HOW TO HELP YOUR FRIEND WITH CANCER

HOW TO HELP YOUR FRIEND WITH CANCER

COLLEEN DOLAN FULLBRIGHT

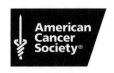

Published by the American Cancer Society/Health Promotion
250 Williams Street NW
Atlanta, Georgia 30303-1002 USA

Printed in the United States of America

Cover design and composition: Rikki Campbell Ogden/pixiedesign llc

Index: Bob Land

5 4 3 2 1   15 16 17 18 19

Library of Congress Cataloging-in-Publication Data

Fullbright, Colleen Dolan.
[Cancer]
How to help your friend with cancer / by Colleen Dolan Fullbright.
pages cm
Revision of: Cancer. 2005.
Includes bibliographical references and index.
ISBN 978-1-60443-224-4 (paperback) — ISBN 1-60443-224-1 (paperback) 1. Cancer—Psychological aspects. 2. Helping behavior. I. Title.
RC262.F86 2014
616.99'4—dc23

     2014030700

AMERICAN CANCER SOCIETY
Managing Director, Content: Chuck Westbrook
Director, Book Publishing: Len Boswell
Managing Editor, Book Publishing: Rebecca Teaff, MA
Senior Editor, Book Publishing: Jill Russell
Coordinator, Book Publishing: Vanika Jordan, MSPub
Editorial Assistant, Book Publishing: Amy Rovere

For more information about cancer, contact your American Cancer Society at **800-227-2345** or **cancer.org**.

Quantity discounts on bulk purchases of this book are available. For information, please contact the American Cancer Society, Health Promotion Publishing, 250 Williams Street NW, Atlanta, GA 30303-1002, or send an e-mail to trade.sales@cancer.org.

FOR ALL WHO BROUGHT
LEVITY AND **LIGHT** TO
MY CANCER EXPERIENCE

CONTENTS

PREFACE

My breast cancer was diagnosed in the fall of 2000. I went through surgery, six months of chemotherapy, and six weeks of radiation therapy. In retrospect, my cancer experience turned out very well. I was fortunate. I had very good medical insurance. I had an excellent oncology team located in the city where I live and was spared long drives for treatment. I was in an ongoing support group for women with breast cancer, and I became close to other members with whom I'm still in contact. My family lived close by and was wonderful.

And I had loyal friends, too. Here's one of my favorite memories: I was newly bald and not at all fond of the wig I'd purchased. My friend took me out to lunch one day and suggested that we stop by Macy's afterward. She wanted to help me find a hat, she said. I stood in the dressing room while she gathered hats for me to try on. I tried on all sorts—whatever she brought in—high fashion, plain, sophisticated, off-the-wall. She tried on a few herself. We giggled a lot. I arrived home with three hats and that warm, splendid feeling one has when you've been the recipient of another's thoughtfulness. Kindness works wonders.

Few generalities can be made about the cancer experience, except that—for most people—it is the scariest time of their lives. It might be the loneliest time, too. Everyone who has cancer needs help from others: practical assistance, emotional support, kind words, and loving gestures.

This book is a compilation of suggestions for how you can provide that help. Whether you have a friend, neighbor, or coworker who is facing cancer, there are ways you can assist her and her loved ones.

I used a variety of sources in the course of my research. Primarily, I talked with other people with cancer and their friends, families, and caregivers about the kinds of help and comfort they found most beneficial. I also contacted researchers and talked with oncology professionals. And I did a lot of reading—books and articles, websites and blogs. Some of the books were academic, and some were not. The websites and blogs were of a diverse mixture—information from cancer organizations or opinion pieces by well-known authors or sites that offered a glimpse into the lives of those dealing with cancer. I sat in on support groups, as well. I found that these visits provided some helpful suggestions from members and affirmed much of what I ran across in the literature: That fatigue is the most common complaint throughout the cancer experience. That people who've had cancer live with the fear of recurrence no matter how long it's been since their treatment. That avoidance by friends is hurtful and difficult to understand.

Many people graciously contributed to this book, some in huge ways. I would like to thank Jennifer Alexander, Amy Wing's Support Group, Nina Bjornsson, John Calderazzo, Marsha Callegari, Peter Callegari, Nancy Campbell, SueEllen Campbell, Pattie Cowell, Brock Dethier, Jim Fullbright, John-Paul Gomez, Melody Graulich, Jeanice Hansen, Luana Heikes, Leonor Kennell, Jean Lamm, Jana Bolduan Lomax, Ann Magennis, Susan Mann, Linda Miller, Sherry Pomering, Dan Robinson, and my dear friend, recording artist Dogwood Daughter. I am deeply indebted to the following people from the American Cancer Society: Jill Russell, my editor, for her gentle guidance and expertise—a joy to work with. Rebecca Teaff and Amy Rovere, for their valuable editorial support. Vanika Jordan, for her many vital contributions as production coordinator. And finally, Len Boswell, director of publishing, to whom I owe a hearty and heartfelt thank you.

There will always be one more idea that was not included in this book. It is my great hope, however, that this book will serve you well as a starting point. Helping one another is such a vital part of human nature.

— *Colleen Dolan Fullbright*

INTRODUCTION

A friend calls to tell you that she has received a diagnosis of ovarian cancer. You can hear the shock and devastation in her voice, and you want to provide some comfort. You have never been at a loss for words, but suddenly, you don't know what to say.

A longtime neighbor recently had surgery for thyroid cancer and will soon begin daily radiation treatments. She is a single mother with an unreliable car. You want to help her but don't have a lot of time. What do you do?

You hear that a friend and longtime coworker has just learned he has colon cancer. You're not sure what to say or do for him. And because he has a large group of friends, you wonder whether he really needs your help.

Shock. Indecision. Helplessness. Fear. When you first learn that a friend has cancer, you might feel some of the same emotions she is experiencing—shock, fear, helplessness. These feelings can make it all the more difficult to know what to do. You may even think about avoiding your friend altogether because of your own discomfort and fear.

Avoidance is not a good idea: she needs you. Though many factors will figure in her recovery, support from friends and family will be crucial—from diagnosis through treatment and into life after treatment. Help and encouragement from family and friends can benefit a person going through cancer in countless ways. Friends can reframe the situation so it feels less overwhelming and threatening. They can lessen their friend's stress by providing emotional support or offering concrete help, such as lending a hand with chores or childcare. Friends can be a welcome distraction and, above all, remind the person that she is valued, loved, and not alone.

Yet many people simply don't know what to do. They want to help but don't want to bother their friend to ask how best to do so. They worry about saying the wrong thing. It can be hard to know how best to support a friend with cancer.

This book is written to give some practical guidance for anyone trying to help a friend or coworker through a difficult experience. The suggestions in these pages will help you support your friend, express your concern, and provide practical assistance. No two people with cancer react in quite the same way to their experience. But all people with cancer have unforeseen needs that only friends and family can meet. Whether you have lots of time or just a little, have a take-charge manner or quiet demeanor, are medically inclined or not, you will have a niche to fill.

It is also important to remember that no two relationships are alike. Different people have different strengths, and we play different roles in each others' lives. Choose the ideas that seem best for your situation. Your choices will depend upon many factors, including your available time, your friend's receptiveness to offers of help, her specific cancer and its treatment, whether she lives nearby or far away, and how close you are to her, her caregiver, and her family. You may find that gender makes a difference, too. In general, men react more stoically to illness than women, whereas women tend to be more open to dialogue.

For clarity and simplicity, I have used "she" and "her" throughout the text to refer to the person with cancer, and "he" and "him" when referring to the caregiver. However, this book is written for people of either gender. Likewise, the ideas found here are not only appropriate for people with cancer, but for anyone dealing with a serious, long-term illness.

You will also see the word *survivor* used at various points throughout the book. The term cancer survivor can refer to anyone who has received a cancer diagnosis, from the time of diagnosis on through the remainder of life. However, some who are living with cancer object to being labeled a survivor. Some feel that it diminishes those who have not survived. Some others object to the wide net cast by the term survivor. Not only does an individual living with cancer fall under this net, but some definitions of a survivor also include the family members, friends, and caregivers of the person with cancer. Each individual has the right to decide how and whether to adopt the term survivor. It is a personal choice and one that is deeply entwined with the person's own experience with cancer.

I have divided the cancer experience into three phases: Diagnosis, During Treatment, and After Treatment Ends. The diagnosis phase lasts from the time that one learns he or she has cancer until treatment begins. The treatment phase could include surgery, chemotherapy, radiation therapy, a bone marrow transplant, other treatments, or a combination of those. In the "after treatment ends" phase, one has completed active treatment but still has a lengthy follow-up period with examinations, tests, and possibly long-term courses of medications. As one progresses through each phase, he or she will experience different emotions, energy levels, and needs. For each phase, I have described some general characteristics and suggested ways you can help your friend. You'll notice there are very few "don'ts" and lots of "do's." There are few hard-and-fast rules.

I've also included some guidance for helping the caregiver and the family. When I think of supporting someone with cancer, I like to think of her "circle," too. She's in the middle, surrounded by a circle of loved ones. All of these loved ones—whether children, a partner or spouse, parents, siblings, or others—will be affected and will be "co-sufferers." They, too, need lots of support and kindness. As writer Terry Tempest Williams (1992) has noted: An individual doesn't get cancer, a family does (p. 214).

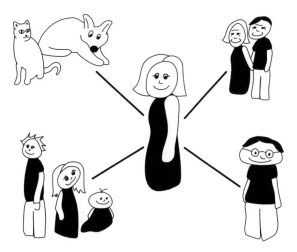

xv

Everyone's circle of loved ones will look a little bit different, of course. The combinations are endless. Mine included my husband; a married daughter with very young children; a son in his senior year of college; my mother, who lived close by; and our beloved cat, K.C. Another's circle might include parents and siblings, or young children and no spouse, or others outside the traditional family circle.

Keep in mind that for the person with cancer, the love and concern will go both ways—she will be concerned about her family, her circle, as much as they are concerned about her. Apprehension about her loved ones may weigh on her. When I had cancer, I worried a great deal about my mother. I remember fearing that my cancer was harder on her than even on me. If your friend has children still at home, she might find it troublesome that she can't do all she normally does for them. She may be anxious about her spouse or partner's stress level. It's difficult not to be able to protect the people we love from worry and suffering, and she may feel guilt or stress that she cannot do all she wants for the people in her circle. Helping to support your friend's loved ones can ease her stress and worry, as well.

Finally, there is a brief section on what to do for your friend if there is no longer hope for a cure for her disease. I hope this is not your situation, but even in that difficult time, there are ways you can support and love your friend.

While I've divided the content into phases, it is important to note that many of the suggestions in the book will apply throughout the person's cancer experience. The person may need more practical assistance during treatment, but she will still need the compassionate ear of her friend, just as she did when her cancer was first diagnosed. She will still need to laugh and be distracted. She will still need to know that her friends are there for her, as they were before this crisis.

As you try to help your friend through this experience, remember to go easy on yourself. Your words may be clumsy at times, and your overtures may feel awkward. Don't worry. When your actions are motivated by love, kindness, and genuine concern, they will be appreciated.

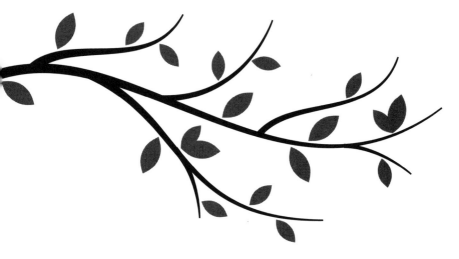

CHAPTER 1

DIAGNOSIS

Fall, 2000: When I received the call from the hospital radiologist telling me that a biopsy had revealed a malignancy in my breast—something about "ductal carcinoma"—it was late on a Friday afternoon and I was home alone. I remember asking the voice on the other end of the line, "Does that mean I have cancer?"

"Yes, I'm afraid so."

"What do I do now?" I asked.

"Well, you'll need to find a surgeon…"

I will never forget that brief conversation. I felt just as I had when a police officer came to the door in 1974 and told me my father was dead. I couldn't take in the words. I didn't know what to do. I hadn't expected that the abnormality on my mammogram would be anything more than a cyst. Like most of us who have gone through cancer, I couldn't have been less prepared for the news. I remember driving frantically over to my mother's house and blurting out to her, "I have cancer!"

In the beginning, when the diagnosis is announced, there is no rational thinking, no plan—just shock. In an instant, the person is thrust into an unfamiliar and frightening world.

From the time that she learns she has cancer until the day she begins treatment, your friend will be faced with major decisions. She may feel rushed to make choices and yet have trouble processing information or recognizing that she has options. She will wonder why this is happening to her. She will wonder whether she is going to die.

At this point, she will need time to absorb what is happening. She will need high-quality, up-to-date information so that she can begin to sort out her options and determine where to go from here. And more than anything, she will need support from friends and loved ones and assurance that they will be there for her throughout her experience.

There are three basic types of support: emotional, instrumental, and informational (Helgeson & Cohen, 1996). *Emotional support* is the verbal and nonverbal communication of caring and concern—

being there, listening, empathizing, comforting. *Instrumental support* includes furnishing material goods or providing a service, such as transportation or housecleaning help—the practical, concrete sort of support. And *informational support* is the provision of information to guide or advise. Some sorts of support are more helpful at different stages than others. In general, though, emotional support is always helpful. Survey after survey bears this out.

It can be difficult just to be with someone without trying to fix things. But sometimes just being there is precisely what is needed. As you think about how best to be there for your friend, remember these words from Henri J. M. Nouwen (1974): "We feel quite uncomfortable with an invitation to enter into someone's pain before doing something about it. Still, when we honestly ask ourselves which persons in our lives mean the most to us, we often find that it is those who, instead of giving much advice, solutions, or cures, have chosen rather to share our pain and touch our wounds with a gentle and tender hand" (p. 38).

Most of the following suggestions will be helpful not only in the period just after diagnosis, but also during your friend's treatment and beyond. In general, try to remember that whatever would be helpful to a healthy person is likely to be beneficial to someone with cancer, unless it also creates additional work or pressure. And remember, little things do count. The right touch, a knowing glance, or a kind smile can do wonders.

3

DO...

GET IN TOUCH WITH HER, and keep in touch.
This may seem basic. But when I sat in on a
support group for those with cancer—many
whose journeys had been long ones, and their
cancers advanced—I learned just how common it
is for friends of people with cancer to disappear.
For these group members, the memory of having
been avoided or abandoned—perhaps years
earlier—was still fresh and still stung.

Stephanie Madsen (2014), a motivational speaker
and three-time cancer survivor, describes cancer as
the adult version of cooties. "Getting it is not cool,
and will send some around you scurrying away in
search of a large tree to hide behind," she writes.
And as hard as it is to understand why friends
flee—it's not as though the person with cancer
doesn't notice—it's a reality that some friendships
do not survive the challenge.

You may be uneasy contacting her the first time
after the diagnosis. This is normal. If words escape
you, you might tell her that you're not quite sure
what to say, but you will be with her throughout
her illness. If you can't visit or live far away, send
cards and notes. Actual physical cards sent through
the mail are especially nice, as your friend can
display them or keep them close by and look at
them over and over again. You might even include
a photo that she'll like. Continue to send cards
and notes throughout her treatment. Many people

tend to send a card only at the beginning of the illness. Don't worry if your message stays the same; a simple "I'm thinking of you" is fine. Leave a supportive voicemail message when you know she will be gone to treatment: extend your good wishes and tell her she doesn't need to call you back.

LET HER TALK. And talk, and talk, if necessary. One of my newly diagnosed friends found that talking about issues with her friends over and over again while they listened was the only way for her to clarify her thoughts. Remember: you are not there to provide medical advice or theological answers. Simply listen. In *Kitchen Table Wisdom: Stories That Heal*, Dr. Rachel Naomi Remen (1997) writes of the power of listening:

5

> *When we interrupt what someone is saying to let them know that we understand, we move the focus of attention to ourselves. When we listen, they know we care. Many people with cancer talk about the relief of having someone just listen.*
>
> *I have even learned to respond to someone crying by just listening. In the old days I used to reach for the tissues, until I realized that passing a person a tissue may be just another way to shut them down, to take them out of their experience of sadness and grief. Now I just listen. When they have cried all they need to cry, they find me there with them.*

This simple thing has not been that easy to learn. It certainly went against everything I had been taught since I was very young. I thought people listened only because they were too timid to speak or did not know the answer. A loving silence often has far more power to heal and to connect than the most well-intentioned words (p. 144).

LET YOUR FRIEND DECIDE what to talk about and with whom. Many well-intentioned friends will attempt to draw their friend out, to encourage her to disclose her deepest thoughts and fears. It is best not to force these types of conversations. Also, do not feel slighted if you offer help and she chooses to draw on others. There are plenty of tasks to go around. We all need to be needed, but let her decide how and with whom to share her concerns.

SIMPLE, HEARTFELT EXPRESSIONS are comforting. Your words needn't be profound. People sometimes feel that if they don't have anything insightful to say, if they can't find the "right" thing to say, they shouldn't say anything at all. Your friend doesn't need profound words; she needs the comfort and presence of someone who cares. And don't be anxious if there are quiet periods when you're together: better silence than hollow words. In fact, silence can be restorative.

BE GENUINE. "Cancer is a disease, not a demand to reinvent a relationship" (p. 176), wrote Dr. Roger Granet (2001) in *Surviving Cancer Emotionally*. Your friend needs the security of knowing you will be the same person with her you have always been. In one survey, a majority of people with cancer felt their family and friends exhibited optimism that felt inauthentic (Peters-Golden, 1982). You can be optimistic, of course, but don't overdo it. Acknowledge her fears, doubts, and concerns; don't downplay them. People with cancer need all types of support from family and friends, not just a cheering section.

BE CALM. Your composure can serve as a source of stability during a time of high anxiety. Try not to become excessively emotional. You can certainly mourn with your friend and express your sorrow, but you want to console her, not the other way around. However, it is important to find someone you can go to for comfort who can be there for you. Perhaps it's your spouse or partner, another friend, or a clergy member. Even a pet can be a source of comfort and calm. The important thing is that you find an outlet for your own feelings.

TRY TO GIVE balanced support. Everyone has times when she needs more space than others, times when a person wants to talk and times when she wants quiet. Try to express your concern for your friend without being intrusive. Give her space without letting her feel deserted. If you're not sure you're striking the right balance, ask her directly how you can best support her. Don't make assumptions. Balance is essential, too, in allowing your friend to feel capable. She's still a competent person; she's just been thrust into an unfamiliar world. Let her do for herself in whatever ways she feels comfortable. Her levels of self-reliance will probably fluctuate during the course of her illness.

BE SENSITIVE to her particular coping style. There are a number of ways that people cope when faced with cancer. Some rely on their faith; others turn to humor. Some people need to vent to friends and family to come to terms with what's happening in their lives. Some people use "problem-focused coping"—they might employ a long-range plan, for example—while others have a more "emotion-focused coping" style—like the use of humor (Gilbar & Ben-Zur, 2002). Usually people draw on a combination of strategies. Counselors emphasize that there is no one "right" way to cope. Accept your friend's coping mechanisms. Be supportive of her own style of expressing her fears, pain, and anger. Don't put your expectations or desires on her. Your job is to be there, listen, and help, not direct or make her feel as if she has to act a certain way.

If she is an extrovert, she will most likely acquire her sense of well-being and resilience from others, according to Jana Bolduan Lomax (personal communication, March 13, 2014), a clinical health psychologist who works in cancer support services. She will likely be more open to frequent visitors than someone who is introverted. Lomax says introverts tend to look within themselves for their strength and rejuvenation, and they will need more privacy and solitude in their cancer journey than extroverts.

Keep in mind you may need to expand your comfort zone just a bit if you are unaccustomed to a particular coping mechanism. Your friend may be angry, for example, and need to vent her anger and frustration as a way to cope. During trying times, keep in mind that your friend has selected you as someone around whom she can safely be herself. Let her.

RESIST THE URGE to change the subject whenever something uncomfortable comes up. In one study, researchers from Virginia Commonwealth University examined supportive and unsupportive behaviors experienced by people with cancer (Grange, Matsuyama, Ingram, Lyckholm, & Smith, 2008). Among other findings, they found that it was important for those with cancer to have people in their social networks who were available and willing to listen to their cancer-related concerns, needs, or stories. When this type of support was absent, there was a strong sense of how valuable it would have been to have people listen to them. People need to feel heard, even if the subject is uncomfortable.

9

RECOGNIZE HOW DIFFICULT IT MAY BE for your friend to ask for and accept help. It is easier for most of us to give than receive. Leslie Wolowitz, a Chicago-based clinical psychologist, has noted that we grow up learning to be "anti-dependent" (Sherman, 2014). The habit of "doing it ourselves" can be hard to let go. Self-reliance and independence are among the toughest things to give up, and, for many of us, needing help can give rise to a scary feeling of vulnerability. You might acknowledge this possibility and tell your friend that she would be giving you a gift in allowing you to help. Express to her that while you cannot make her well, you want—and need—to support her.

OFFER TO HELP, and don't stop with the initial offer. At the outset, she may believe that she can handle everything by herself. As treatment progresses, however, she will realize that she has some limitations. As time passes, she may be more likely to accept assistance. Ask about her needs throughout her illness, even if she says all is well.

When you make offers, propose ideas that fit your time and abilities. Don't offer to drive if traffic makes you crazy or offer to cook if you always burn the oatmeal. Jeanice Hansen (personal communication, March 13, 2014), an oncology social worker at Saint Joseph Hospital Comprehensive Cancer Center in Denver, Colorado, suggests that you say to your friend, "This is what I'm good at and what I like to do."

For example, "I really love to garden. Can I help do the planting? Can I come and pull weeds?" Or, "I can offer my husband. He can come and mow your lawn every Saturday." In this way, you're matching your abilities and your strengths with your friend's needs. When her cancer is first diagnosed, she may not have a good idea of what her schedule will be like. But even at this early stage, you may be able to commit to a regular task. Caring for her pet, for example, taking out the garbage on trash days, or picking up her child from school—these could all be valuable ways to help out. Knowing that she can count on consistent help can lessen her worries a bit and help her and her family make plans. Keep in mind that you will need to follow through with whatever you put forward.

BE SPECIFIC in your offers. Say, "I would like to do/tell/find _____." A vague "let me know if you need any help," while well intentioned, is not helpful. Chances are high that she won't let you know, or she won't have the time or energy to identify her needs and call you to ask for help. Try to be specific and concrete. Some further examples of ways to help follow, and many more can be found in the next section, "During Treatment."

FIND RELIABLE INFORMATION, if she asks for it. The need for trustworthy information is one of the top concerns of new patients and their caregivers (Matthews, Baker, & Spillers, 2004). Doctors

11

sometimes do not fulfill this need adequately because they underestimate their patients' capabilities to understand the complexities of treatment options (Keitel & Kopala, 2000). At diagnosis, your friend will likely feel as though she is in a whirlwind and can't quite get her bearings. This might especially be true in finding information. Ask her what types of information she needs. Would she like to know more about her specific type of cancer? Information about doctors or specific treatments?

There are some caveats to consider. There are many websites where you can find all types of information on cancer, treatment options, clinical trials, and complementary and alternative treatments. But because anyone can post information online, it's important to evaluate all sources carefully. For example, what type of organization is publishing the information? In the United States, the most reputable sources tend to be government agencies, hospitals, universities, and major public health organizations. These types of entities will publish information that has been reviewed by experts and will update that information often. In general, beware of sites that promise scientific breakthroughs, miracle cures, or that a product can cure a wide range of illnesses (American Cancer Society, 2014). The American Cancer Society offers more information on its website about sorting through cancer information on the Internet.

OFFER TO FIND OTHER CANCER SURVIVORS with the same diagnosis, if she is open to the idea. Psychooncologists have found that people who have been through cancer—"veteran patients"—are better equipped to understand the patient's concerns, especially in areas that might be hard to talk about with family members (Mastrovito, Moynihan, & Parsonnet, 1989). For example, someone facing a loss of bowel function or a change in sexual capabilities may depend desperately upon other people who have been through similar experiences for reassurance. It might be easier for a person with cancer to trust a veteran patient to hear her honest thoughts, feelings, and concerns without judgment or disappointment. Talk with someone at a hospital, clinic, or local agency about finding a veteran patient to support your friend. A support group also might be helpful for her (see the next point).

HELP HER FIND A SUPPORT GROUP, if she feels that she might benefit from one. In a similar vein to the point above, many people are helped by talking with a group of people going through similar experiences. A support group can help dispel myths, provide support and information, and serve as an outlet for feelings that might be difficult to share with healthy friends or family. If she does attend a group, offer to drive her there and back. Most oncology clinics offer support groups for their patients. In addition, the

13

American Cancer Society offers links to online support through its website (go to cancer.org and click on "Find Support & Treatment"). These include sites such as the American Cancer Society Cancer Survivors Network® (csn.cancer.org). See the resource guide at the back of this book for other websites that might be helpful.

OFFER TO GO WITH HER to her medical appointments and take notes. Note-taking by someone other than the person with cancer is crucial. Take on the role of Chief Scribe for her. You might even record the sessions, if possible. Most newly diagnosed people—perhaps still somewhat in shock—forget much of what they've been told by their doctors. After diagnosis, she may have to undergo a number of tests—bone scans, MRIs, and other tests—some of which can be lengthy and stressful. It may be that her spouse or caregiver wants to go with her to appointments but sometimes has to attend to other obligations—such as work or caring for the children. He is likely juggling lots of responsibilities, and going with your friend would be of help to him, too.

IF YOU SHARE THE SAME FAITH or religious traditions, you might encourage her in that way, or share in religious practices or rituals with her. If your friend is religious or spiritual and you share in these beliefs, nurturing that spirituality

14

is one way you can support her. Maintaining a sense of the spiritual in one's life can make a huge difference, particularly in a stressful or difficult time. Dr. C. M. Puchalski (2012), in her research, has found that spirituality can have an impact on how a person deals with her illness, gets meaning out of the experience, and can affect her concept of health and quality of life. It can help in promoting a sense of wellness, even while she is dealing with the challenges of cancer and its treatment. For many people with cancer, their spirituality helps them cope and make sense of what's happening, as well as enabling them to find meaning in their lives.

DON'T...

DON'T TELL YOUR FRIEND about others who had cancer and did not survive! Although it seems hard to believe, people with cancer often report hearing these sorts of stories from friends. It is not a good morale booster. It also might be wise not to try to create too much optimism by telling "success stories." Overall, less is more.

DON'T SUGGEST that a positive attitude alone will cure her. Joanie Willis and her coauthors (2001) write in the book, *The Cancer Patient's Workbook*: "Attitude CANNOT override biology. Biology is biology is biology" (p. 109). This does

15

not mean that hope and a positive outlook are not vital. However, a particular outlook will not be the sole determinant in the outcome of any cancer experience. Unknowingly, some friends and family may put pressure on the person with cancer to be positive at all costs. In *Patients With Cancer: Understanding the Psychological Pain*, Arlene Houldin (2000) cautions that "well-intentioned advice [from family and friends] may take the form of demands that the cancer patient must be the exceptional patient—one who is unwaveringly positive, always fighting the disease, never showing any negative emotion... The fundamental problem with this line of thinking is that the *exceptional patient is fictional*" (p. 2–3).

Other cancer survivors have described similar experiences. Arthur Frank (2002), in *At the Will of the Body: Reflections on Illness*, speaks of the cost of trying to sustain an unfailingly positive image, as well as feeling pressure from those around him to embody that cheerful, strong persona: "[It] cost me energy, which was scarce. It also cost me opportunities to express what was happening in my life with cancer and to understand that life. Finally, my attempts at a positive image diminished my relationships with others by preventing them from sharing my experience" (p. 67).

It is good to be positive, of course. But your friend's future does not depend on it.

DON'T SPECULATE about what might have caused her cancer. This type of speculation really serves no purpose.

DON'T "PITY" HER. Remember the difference between pity and empathy. Pity is to feel sorry for someone, and it can come across as condescending and unhelpful. Empathy, however, means that you are trying to sense in part what your friend is going through.

DON'T TELL HER how to feel. Statements such as "you should feel lucky that they found it when they did" or "there's nothing to be afraid of" can feel patronizing or even uncaring. Telling her to cheer up may well annoy her, understandably. She needs her friends to acknowledge her fears, not dismiss them. Similarly, don't say, "I know just what you're going through." Acknowledge your own fear without dwelling on it, but don't say that you know how she feels. You don't. Simply saying, "I'm scared sometimes, too," might do.

AVOID CLICHÉS. Your intentions might be good when you want to tell your friend to keep fighting or that you admire her bravery. But for many people living with cancer, the cliché of cancer as a battle to be won is not appropriate. Not everyone wants to be a fighter or be admired: they simply want to live their lives.

17

DON'T TREAT HER like a "cancer patient." She is not her disease. Try to remember to just treat her like your friend. Cancer is not contagious.

DON'T MAKE ASSUMPTIONS about her faith and practices. As discussed earlier, a spiritual presence in one's life can be beneficial and life-affirming. If you want to offer your friend spiritual support, however, be very thoughtful about what you offer. Jeanice Hansen (personal communication, March 13, 2014) notes that while many religious communities encourage their members to witness their faith to others, it may not be received as helpful if the person does not share your beliefs. She suggests that you ask permission before you make an overture. "You might ask, 'Would it be all right if I pray for you?' We each have different ways of coping with life's challenges. When it comes to relying on our religious faith, spiritual beliefs, or existential views, we need to be respectful of these differences—and commonalities—as well."

CHAPTER 2

DURING
TREATMENT

What to say about my own cancer treatment? It was standard for breast cancer with lymph node involvement: surgery, chemotherapy, radiation therapy. It went extraordinarily well.

At the same time, it was no picnic. Some days I found humor in my situation; other days I could see nothing funny anywhere. Sometimes, chemotherapy went so slowly that I could practically count, one by one, the drops of chemicals going into my body through the port in my chest. It was unbelievingly boring. Other times, I was engaged in such lively conversation with strangers, all of us sharing a common experience in the chemo room, that I didn't want it to end.

My treatment went well, but for some of my fellow patients, it was not all smooth sailing. The anti-nausea drugs I was given worked well for me. Others suffered severe nausea after chemotherapy, despite taking medication to prevent it. My blood counts stayed pretty stable, assuring me that I could go on with my chemotherapy as scheduled. Others experienced low white blood cell counts that meant they had to postpone treatments to let their bodies recover. I think it must be hard to predict who will suffer serious side effects from the treatment and who will breeze right through. I guess maybe it's a matter of luck, and I was on the lucky side.

Your friend's treatment may involve surgery, radiation therapy, chemotherapy, or a combination of these. Depending on her circumstances, a bone marrow transplant may be necessary. Your friend could have many side effects or very few. She could experience nausea or vomiting, pain, hair loss, appetite or weight changes, mouth sores, or skin problems. She will likely experience fatigue and depleted energy levels. She may have trouble concentrating or have trouble with her memory. The regular, everyday chores and tasks of life may be too much for her to accomplish without help.

Questions about the meaning of life and the prospect of death—an "existential plight"—usually surface now. Psychiatrists A. D. Weisman and J. W. Worden (1976–1977) note that these issues begin at diagnosis and generally manifest most during the first one hundred days following diagnosis. It often takes this long for cancer patients to realize the seriousness of their illness.

Your friend might be troubled by an urgent desire to get things done. A source of anxiety for many people with cancer is the sense of time running out. According to psychologist Robert Chernin Cantor (1978), the person may envision his or her lifetime as beginning to shrink. "Attention shifts to the immediate future. The thought of fulfilling all one's needs, the idea of completing all the unrealized projects of a lifetime, can be overwhelming" (p. 223).

A person going through cancer treatment experiences "secondary losses." She is not only losing her good health, but also her sense of control and her sense of life's predictability. She may lose her job and financial security. She may lose her hair and her eyebrows. Your friend may struggle with these physical changes and with letting go of these parts of her life, even if the losses are temporary. It may feel like cancer has changed everything, and the awareness of these losses can hit hard in this phase.

It is essential that your friend be able to grieve. Grieving is an important way for people with

21

cancer to mourn these very real losses and find new purpose. Be available to listen—a lot. You do not need to have a solution for her losses; sometimes there aren't any solutions.

Your friend may also struggle with the conflict between an intensified dependence on others and a desire for more independence. It's helpful to remember that this is an unavoidable part of the cancer experience. Dr. Julia Rowland (1989) writes that "[f]or both patient and caretaker, there may be bad feelings about having to be 'cared for' and 'caring for'" (p. 36). This is especially true if either's role has changed significantly as a result of the cancer.

If your friend has children at home, their needs will be vital. Active treatment can take many months, and she will want to keep her children's lives as normal as possible. Although some disruption is unavoidable, her children need to keep to their usual routines, with loving and familiar people around them. For suggestions on how to help a friend who has children at home, see "Supporting the Family and Caregiver," beginning on page 41.

As you read the suggestions in the following pages, keep in mind that some of the help you offer could require a major commitment of your time. You will need to follow through. Also, many of the suggestions in this section could be carried out in conjunction with others—members of your church, coworkers, neighbors, or friends. If you

22

would like to pay for regular housecleaning for your friend, for example, but could not afford the cost by yourself, maybe you could recruit others to pitch in. Maybe several of you could work together to provide meals for your friend and her family. There are times when having cancer seems outside the realm of life as most of us know it. For a person going through cancer treatment, "normal" life has been put on hold. Friends who can recognize this fact can help make life as normal as possible, in addition to just being there and supporting her as she faces the challenges of cancer treatment.

DO...

REMEMBER that even if your friend already has a strong social network, she will still need you. Support—and even contact—often drops off as time goes on. Many people with cancer find that the enthusiastic overtures of support and gestures of affection they received at diagnosis fade some during treatment. In one study, over half of those with cancer felt that they had been avoided or feared (Peters-Golden, 1982). In their book, *Reclaiming Your Life After Diagnosis*, Kim Thiboldeaux and Dr. Mitch Golant (2012) describe how friends sometimes find it hard to see someone they care about suffer. Some people feel helpless and struggle to know how to help. For others, there can even be a fear, however

23

irrational, that cancer is contagious. Don't assume that your support is unimportant because she has other friends. They may not be as involved as you think. As far as friends go, the more, the better.

CALL BEFORE YOU VISIT. Though your friend needs contact with her comrades, she will not always be up for visitors. Treatment can be exhausting, and you will want to be sure that you drop by at a time that's convenient and welcome. When you do visit, greet her as you always have, with a hug or a smile. Her appearance may have changed as a result of the cancer or the treatments. Try not to express alarm. And don't put her in the awkward position of having to comfort you.

BE SENSITIVE to times she may need rest or time alone. At times, your friend may be worn out and simply need rest. Time alone may feel like a relief at times—a welcome interval when she doesn't have to attend so much to the feelings of those around her. Many, however, have difficulty expressing this need to their friends and loved ones. In the book *What Helped Get Me Through: Cancer Survivors Share Wisdom and Hope* (Silver, 2009), cancer survivors were asked what would have helped them, had they felt able to ask for it. One respondent wrote, "To be left alone" (p. 237). Another said, "Admitting to others that I didn't feel well and needed more rest" (p. 239). When I spoke with Jeanice Hansen (personal communication, March 13, 2014), the oncology social worker at Saint Joseph Hospital in Denver, she explained how she teaches her patients to voice their needs. But not everyone gets training like this, and some people will find it difficult to speak up. You could be helpful in being sensitive to her needs without her needing to voice them.

ALLOW HER SOME LEEWAY in her social skills. One of my friends who faced cancer described the experience of being a cancer patient as being in a different world, one an outsider could not understand. Don't be offended if the "normal" rules regarding courtesies, thanks, or responses do not always seem to apply. Be aware that she will have good days and bad days, and occasional expressions of negativity and anger are normal reactions to the illness.

REALIZE THAT SHE WILL WANT to hear about subjects other than her illness. Talk with her about current events, sports, bestsellers, your family—whatever you would normally talk about. However, don't avoid talking about the cancer. Pretending it's not there will not make it go away. It can sometimes be difficult to find the right balance, and her needs may vary from day to day.

OFFER TO BE HER CHAUFFEUR. In general, transportation is a paramount concern for people undergoing cancer treatment (Matthews, Baker, &

25

Spillers, 2004), and lack of transportation can be a huge barrier to receiving high-quality care (Institute of Medicine Committee on Psychosocial Services to Cancer Patients, 2008). There might be times when your friend does not have enough energy to drive to an appointment or get out for fresh air, and she will likely have many appointments, medical and otherwise. Radiation therapy, for example, can require treatment every weekday for a period of weeks. If she has a spouse or primary caregiver, that person might have other work or family obligations that make it difficult to be the sole provider of transportation. If you have transportation and some flexibility in your schedule, offer to help. Keep in mind that these appointments could be very important parts of her treatment, and she will be counting on you. You'll really need to follow through. If you are personally unable to provide transportation but discover that she needs help getting to appointments, contact the American Cancer Society at 800-227-2345 to find out whether they have programs in your community to help transport people to appointments. For more information on organizations that can assist with transportation, see the resource guide starting on page 79.

SIT WITH HER at chemotherapy or other appointments. Cancer can be lonely—and boring. Chemotherapy treatments can last for hours, and waiting for tests can take lots of

26

time. Having a friend with you at times like this is a great distraction. Your friend will appreciate "instrumental support," of course—transportation, help with household tasks, etc.—but, remember, emotional support is the most valuable of all. Your presence alone is a gift.

OFFER TO BE an unofficial "press agent" by assisting with phone calls or e-mail updates for friends and family. She needs to focus on herself and not worry about getting messages to others about her family and current treatment status. There are many websites (such as www.caringbridge.org and www.mylifeline.org) that can help family and friends get updates for a loved one undergoing cancer treatment.

27

GO WITH HER to a wig shop (if she wants to wear a wig) or go shopping for hats with her, if she will be losing her hair from treatment. Few who have lost their hair would enjoy going to a wig salon or standing bald and alone in a department store trying on hats. Trying on wigs and hats can actually be kind of fun, if you have a friend along.

HELP WITH HOUSEWORK or pay someone to do her housecleaning. Your friend may not feel well enough or have the energy to keep up with regular household tasks during treatment. However, many people are too embarrassed to ask for help cleaning their house, even if that is what is needed the most. Help clean her house or, if you can afford it, pay a housecleaner to come periodically. Offer to do her laundry or change the sheets on her bed, if she is comfortable with that. These simple household tasks can be very meaningful.

BRING MEALS or help coordinate efforts among friends. When you think about keeping a household running smoothly, your first thought is likely food. It's a daily necessity. Dishes that can be frozen and reheated later, such as precooked casseroles, lasagna, and macaroni and cheese, are usually the most convenient. (If she has children at home, bringing over take-out might be helpful and more appealing for kids than something thawed and reheated.) You might enlist other friends to commit to certain days so that each day is covered. People sometimes create "meal trains," in which friends and neighbors work together to ensure meal coverage. There are even websites one can use to enable people to sign up for days and meals. If you are coordinating meal delivery, try to set times for deliveries so that your friend and her family know what to expect. Put the food in disposable containers so that dishes do not have to be returned. Be sure to ask about any special dietary needs and communicate this information to the people participating. Some treatments cause mouth sores or other impediments to eating, and many chemotherapy drugs cause nausea or aversions to certain foods. It might be helpful to list the ingredients you used if you bring something homemade. Remember that even if your friend can't eat it, her family will enjoy your effort.

If you're not part of providing meals, you might help keep her refrigerator and pantry stocked with essentials. These could include canned or packaged soups and convenient foods, such as canned salmon or tuna, canned beans, and jars of peanut butter. You could help keep her stock of frozen and refrigerated food organized, especially if lots of people are bringing meals. You also could check that the refrigerator is cleaned out regularly.

OFFER TO DO YARD WORK—mowing and watering the lawn, shoveling the sidewalks, putting on storm windows—whatever the season requires. One woman going through treatment asked for bedding plants, which her friend promptly purchased, delivered, and planted. Or help with auto maintenance—wash the car, change the oil, or just make sure she has a full tank.

CARE FOR HER PETS. Pets often play a vital role in our lives, and the demands and physical side effects of treatment can mean the person might not have the time she would like to devote to her pet. Offer to pick up their food from the store and keep them fed, take them for walks, clean the cat's litter box, or take them to the vet. Endure her dog's sloppy kisses!

29

CARE FOR HER indoor plants. Some of us have plants that we have nurtured for years. If this is something your friend might appreciate and you have a green thumb, volunteer to look after her plants. If needed, you could have her give you the basics as to frequency and amount of watering and any other instructions.

HELP WITH HOLIDAYS. This can include putting up or taking down a Christmas tree, shopping for gifts, handing out Halloween candy, planning a Fourth of July barbecue, or having a birthday get-together. Holidays can be especially important if your friend has young children. Whatever your friend's normal traditions are, help her do those things. Carrying on special rituals or traditions can help keep the family anchored and bring a sense of normalcy when life seems anything but normal.

HELP HER GET ORGANIZED. Going through cancer treatment can create quite a paper trail. Bills, statements from insurance, correspondence: even for someone who is normally very organized, dealing with this mountain of paperwork while going through treatment is difficult. If you are good at organizing or knowledgeable about insurance, offer to help with the paperwork pertaining to her cancer treatment. Cancer survivor Diane Sims Roth (2003) touches on this very topic in her book *An Ovarian Cancer Companion*: "Chances are that my bills are a

30

pile of unorganized paperwork… I would be enormously grateful if you would come by some day, without judgment as to what kind of mess I have made of the pile, and help me straighten it out. Maybe make a few phone calls. Maybe write a few letters. You wouldn't believe what a difference it would make" (p. 130–131).

HELP HER WRITE THANK-YOU NOTES, or simply mail them for her. Your friend needs to be able to focus on resting and getting through treatment. If she is feeling overwhelmed by the need to thank people for their kindnesses, offer to help share that burden.

GIVE HER A GIFT CERTIFICATE or gift card— for a restaurant (maybe one that offers delivery service), a movie rental service or store, a bookstore, or even a grocery store or gas station. A gift that provides an entertaining diversion, such as movie tickets, a DVD, or a good book, is another good possibility.

31

GIVE HER FINANCIAL ASSISTANCE, if she's in need and you are in the position to help her. Financial aid is difficult to ask for. In the book *What Helped Get Me Through: Cancer Survivors Share Wisdom and Hope* (Silver, 2009), participants were asked what would have helped them, had they felt comfortable asking for it. Many answered with "money" or "financial help."

Cancer can have a devastating impact on a family's finances. In a large survey of U.S. families in which a member of the household had cancer in the past five years, 13 percent had to borrow money to pay for bills, and 10 percent were unable to pay for basic necessities such as food, heat, or housing. In those families without health insurance, more than one in four delayed or decided not to get treatment because of its cost (The Henry J. Kaiser Family Foundation, Harvard School of Public Health, & *USA Today*, 2006).

If you would like to offer financial help, try to be direct but tactful. Try to do so in a way that doesn't make her feel ashamed or embarrassed. Another possibility would be to tell her you'd like to give her a gift by paying for daycare, a regular cleaning service, or another service that would be useful for her. You could purchase a prepaid debit card for her, so that she can use it in whatever way she needs. There are a number of websites that allow people to donate money to help cover expenses. If she is reluctant to look into these types of sites, you could offer to do it.

Some agencies, public and private, offer financial help. See the resource guide beginning on page 79 for information on agencies that offer financial assistance. If it's overwhelming for your friend to sift through the information, offer to look through it to find any that could be pertinent to her situation.

HELP WITH HER ongoing responsibilities and commitments. Depending on your friend's circumstances, this could be an extensive undertaking or a major commitment. One of the frustrating parts of cancer, especially while going through treatment, is that the "outside world" still goes on and the person with cancer's responsibilities are still there. She might be a caregiver for an elderly parent or have important responsibilities at her church, synagogue, or her child's school. If you have adequate free time, consider offering to lend a hand.

GIVE HER SOMETHING personal. Make something if you are so inclined. A friend of mine stitched a pretty scarf for a friend who had lost her hair—a very special gift that was not extremely time-consuming or expensive. Give your friend a poem you love, homemade cards your children made for her, or a batch of homemade cookies.

DO SOMETHING FUN together. This would depend, of course, upon her energy level, but there are many ways you can enjoy time together. Go to a hardware store for a nail to hang that painting, go out to eat, go to a matinee—these can be a welcome change of pace for someone going through cancer treatment. Enjoy some quiet time together outdoors. It doesn't need to be fancy; just set up a couple of chairs. Take a walk. Pack a basket

33

and take her for a picnic. Watch a DVD with her or, if she's a sports fan, watch a game with her on television. Sometimes she will need company but not want to talk. If you participated in activities together before her diagnosis, keep her involved as much as she is able now. Don't exclude her from your everyday life.

OFFER TO GET BOOKS or audiobooks for her from the library, if she likes to read. Don't forget to return them, too! If she doesn't have a portable music player with earphones, buy or loan her one. Or she might appreciate your reading to her. Give her some relaxation CDs. Many find classical music soothing. If she likes movies, pick up and return a couple of DVDs for her.

34

SPEND THE NIGHT WITH HER, or the weekend, if she's alone and would like some company. If she's home alone, company might be a welcome comfort.

HELP EASE her physical discomfort. If she has lost her hair, her scalp may be very tender. New, soft bed linens or a fluffy pillow might be welcome. I read about a woman who gave her friend a new bed! Give her warm socks if it's cold outside or an electric fan for when it's hot. If you're both comfortable with it, you could rub her feet or apply lotion to her hands. Something as simple as smoothing out her sheets and bedcovers can be a big help.

HELP MAKE HER SURROUNDINGS pleasant.
Candles (unscented might be best), a framed
photo of the two of you, new bathroom towels,
a pretty throw blanket, new pillowcases—any of
these show her you're thinking of her. Or give her
a fancy nightgown or nice lounge clothes—these
can help her be comfortable and lift her spirits.
Men and women, of course, may have different
preferences. My friend John chuckled at these
suggestions. "Just give me ESPN," he said. Think
about your friend's personality. When in doubt,
ask around for what may seem right.

**IF AND WHEN YOUR FRIEND IS HOSPITALIZED,
ask her family how you can help.** Being in the
hospital will present its own set of challenges,
both for your friend and her family. A fellow cancer
patient found that his neediest time was when he
was coming out of anesthesia after surgery. "That's
when I most needed moral and practical support,"
he said. He found his friend's presence at his
bedside after surgery immensely comforting. There
might be ways in which you can help the family, as
well, during these challenging times. You might be
the "go-fer" while your friend's family stays with
her, or you might be able to stay with your friend
while the family goes home for a night's rest or
shower and change of clothes. If she has out-of-
town guests, you might offer to have them stay
with you or provide transportation around town or
to and from the airport. You will be helping your
friend by helping her loved ones.

35

DON'T...

DON'T BE AFRAID to touch her. Human touch is a vital need. It provides physical benefits, lowering stress hormones, improving the immune system, lowering blood pressure, and even reducing pain. But more than that, it is a strong means of connection, a simple but profound way to express affection.

DON'T BE AFRAID to laugh with her. Everyone—especially your friend—knows that cancer is a very serious disease. We do not want to make light of it. But just as with touch, laughter provides not only physical benefits—like relief of tension—but is a universal balm in times of distress.

DON'T QUESTION her treatment plan, and don't push things on her (such as alternative treatments you've heard about). In an effort to be helpful, some friends, acquaintances, and family members may share stories they've heard of other people's success stories or new alternative treatments. Try to be respectful of her decisions and her doctors' expertise.

DON'T MAKE NEGATIVE (or inauthentically positive) comments about her appearance. Weight loss, puffiness from steroids, hair loss, fatigue, physical manifestations of surgery: these are all possible side effects from the very treatment aimed at helping your friend get better. Smile when you first see her. But beware of "false cheerfulness," too. You may think that "You look great!" would be a compliment. But as patients in treatment, we know we don't look so great.

AVOID PITY. In a study identifying behaviors that were supportive and not supportive of people going through cancer, participants said they wanted help but did not want to feel that they were being pitied (Grange, Matsuyama, Ingram, Lyckholm, & Smith, 2008). Some people would rather be alone than be pitied (Sprah & Sostaric, 2004). Author Christine Longaker (1997), a pioneer in the hospice movement in the United States, describes the need felt by many going through cancer: to be seen as "a whole person, not as a disease, or a tragedy, or a fragile piece of glass. Do not look at me with pity but rather with all of your love and compassion" (p. 17).

37

IN THE WORKPLACE

Perhaps your friend is your coworker. While she's off work to deal with cancer, here are some ideas on ways to ease her distress:

Volunteer to be the "point person" between her and others in the office who may be sharing in her workload while she's out. If you work closely with her, you may be able to act as the liaison. If you have some advance warning, try to find out what critical items she is handling and the status of any projects. Make sure you have adequate information to represent her in her absence. In addition, it's wise to think about how she wants her absence explained to others outside of (or inside) the organization. Keep in mind that this commitment could last quite some time, so volunteer only if you are sure you can commit for the long haul (Cosmetic Executive Women Foundation, 2014).

Ask her how she'd like to keep in touch if you have work-related questions. If you need to talk with her about workplace matters, she might prefer e-mail to phone calls. If you will need to communicate frequently, arrange how best to do that: a weekly e-mail or phone call, for example. Keep a list of questions or issues that need to be discussed so that they aren't trickling or flooding in. This approach will minimize her stress.

Be sensitive in talking with others about your friend or coworker. There might be issues of confidentiality. Your friend may want to keep some aspects of her cancer private. So make sure to ask her what she'd like to be shared. Be sure that you disclose only as much or as little as she desires.

Donate some of your annual leave or sick leave time to your coworker. Many workplaces have programs in place to allow employees to donate unused annual leave or sick days. This may work differently in different companies, but it is worth investigating. Speak with your human resources representative to find out whether your company offers this benefit.

Help keep coworkers in the loop or coordinate sending cards, flowers, or gifts. Your friend will appreciate something that shows her coworkers are thinking about her. Consider coordinating a gift (such as a gift certificate) or a card from those in the office.

39

Let your ill coworker know, through your actions and words, that she is still part of the team. Much of her identity may be connected to her job. This major disruption may have generated a substantial feeling of loss. Keep her apprised of happenings in the office. Let her know how much she's missed and that her absence is felt. (But be careful not to cause guilt that she's not there to handle the job.)

Give her leeway upon her return. Many who've had cancer feel a need to return to work before they are completely ready or while their energy levels are still very low. It's difficult for some people to resume their duties full-time. Depending on how closely you work with her and what assistance you provided in her absence, you may be able to help your friend ease back into her duties.

40

CHAPTER 3

SUPPORTING
THE FAMILY AND
CAREGIVER

I think our next-door neighbor, Marilyn, had a sixth sense. On the days we needed it most, when treatment seemed to hit me the hardest, we'd hear a knock on the door, and there—out of the blue—would stand Marilyn, with a fabulous casserole or Crock-Pot stew she'd made for us. Oh, how it hit the spot on cold, wintry evenings! Not only did she provide a lovely little respite from cooking, but her thoughtfulness helped remind us that she—and many others—were "with us" on this journey. We weren't going it alone.

Cancer can be a major destabilizer in families (Rait & Lederberg, 1989). Because the stress on family members can sometimes be as great as or greater than that experienced by the person with cancer, psychologists often call family members "second-order patients." Cancer brings about a huge disruption in the roles and routines of the family. A family member often takes on the task of primary caregiving, a role that can be overwhelming. Careers are disrupted. Finances may dwindle. Children lose a particular stability that existed before diagnosis. Fulfilling the daily needs of each individual family member is not always possible, and some members will feel short-changed.

Changes in health care have led to an increase in the amount of hands-on care required at home, meaning the caregiver must take on even more responsibility than in the past. Many treatments that were once done in the hospital are now done on an outpatient basis, and, even if the person is in the hospital, his or her hospitalization time will be shorter, as compared with that of previous years. Many caregivers are expected to carry out demanding and sometimes complicated tasks for which they have no training. The level of psychological, physical, and technical support currently required of caregivers has never been seen before.

The needs of the caregiver frequently go unvoiced and overlooked. He may try hard to remain quiet about his own distress for fear of adding to the tremendous stress and anxiety already present in the family. Research has shown that across the cancer landscape, caregivers may experience levels of psychological stress that are equal to or greater than those of the survivor (Northouse, Mood, Templin, Mellon, & George, 2000). Many caregivers experience a lengthy isolation, as they deal with the demands of caregiving and find that friends no longer keep in touch. Some lose their jobs and lose their "place" in life. The extra demands and cumulative stresses upon the caregiver can become so taxing that some suffer total burnout (Montada, Filipp, & Lerner, 1992). Researchers have found that even two years after the cancer diagnosis, caregivers were still spending an average of eight hours a day providing care (Yabroff & Kim, 2009).

43

Just like the people for whom they are caring, caregivers will have their own ways of coping. Some will handle the tremendous tasks required of them quite smoothly, while others will need more outside help. Those who do need more help must be reassured that this is **not** a sign of weakness. Some will become overprotective in their role and experience great difficulty letting go and letting others help. This may relate to a strong sense of responsibility or a need to feel in control of their own lives, as well as the patient's life.

Caregivers almost always feel guilt at one time or another. They may believe that they aren't doing enough for the person with cancer or feel selfish when they take time for themselves. In some cases, they might believe that they themselves caused the cancer. Some caregivers begin to feel resentful at being trapped in a difficult situation in which there seems to be no light at the end of the tunnel. Friends may perceive the caregiver as overly self-sacrificing and might attempt— with good intentions—to help him look out for himself. This could present a dilemma regarding personal boundaries. I spoke with one woman— her husband's primary caregiver—who found that others' attempts to help her and offer advice tended to undermine her confidence in herself. "There's a tendency," she said, "for others to see this as a time to 'intervene'…Caregivers really are susceptible to assuming (usually wrongly) that others know more about what will 'work' or not than the caregiver herself." Just as you will avoid being patronizing toward your friend, you will also want to avoid that position with her caregiver.

While your friend with cancer is actively engaged in getting better, her other family members will often feel helpless. They may feel that they don't know what's going on or they may have no way to relieve their own anxiety. They frequently feel that they are not entitled to negative feelings and that they should simply try to be positive. Many times family members feel neglected but don't want to voice what they regard as selfish concerns. They feel obliged to focus solely on the person with cancer.

In the book *And a Time to Live*, Robert Chernin Cantor (1978) tells of the director of a suicide prevention center who said he received few calls from people with cancer. Instead, he said, most cancer-related calls came from spouses and relatives. It is not uncommon for the partner of someone with cancer to experience the same level of anxiety and depression as the patient herself. Stress is exacerbated when both partners hold in their emotions for fear of upsetting the other.

A parent's serious illness can affect a child in a profound way. Changes in family routine, such as bedtime rituals and meal times, are especially hard on children, who need the security of a normal schedule in the midst of cancer chaos. Behavior at home and within the family, school performance, mental health, friendships, growth and development—all of these can be affected in real and tangible ways.

Children of all ages will be scared and will react in a variety of ways. Children between three and six years of age fear, above all, separation from their parents. Those between seven and ten are most likely to feel sadness, loneliness, and worry about their family's safety. Between ten and thirteen, children tend to focus on the disruption in their own lives brought about by a parent's illness (Burton, 1998).

Teenagers are particularly affected by the illness and torn by conflicting inclinations.

Developmentally, gradual separation from the family is normal for teenagers, but the illness beckons them back. Often, they will act out or seem apathetic, and they are **not** likely to be positive, loving, or even helpful during the crisis. They need more time off from the family than other members, and they also need more space and privacy. At the same time, however, they need strong support from family and close friends. Being supportive while enduring a teenager's rather unbecoming behavior can be hard, as it is in any family with a teenager in the house! It may require extra patience and flexibility from everyone.

Children of all ages need to feel needed and that they are integral parts of the family. Their contributions in keeping the household going are important for their sense of worth and control. But beware of placing undue expectations upon them. Also, it is vital they be informed and regularly updated, at an age-appropriate level, about the status of the cancer. In the case of children and teenagers, the communication process will be ongoing, not a one-time event (Eyre, Lange, & Morris, 2002).

Dr. Roger Granet (2001) writes, in *Surviving Cancer Emotionally*, "For too long, medical professionals treating the disease have tended to consider family and friends as little more than the backdrop against which cancer's drama played out. Now we are coming to understand that they, too, are profoundly affected by the disease and as needy of attention and care as the patient" (p. 169).

Though it could be seen as secondary, one of the best ways to help your friend is to help her family. I once asked members of a support group about gestures that were especially helpful from friends. One woman emphasized repeatedly how much she had appreciated friends and relatives who brought meals so that her husband would not have to worry about cooking, in addition to taking care of her. It was at the top of her list of things she needed most. When her friends considered her husband's needs, they were demonstrating their love and support for her, too.

Many of the suggestions for supporting your friend also can be used to support your friend's family.

47

DO...

VOLUNTEER TO BE THE POINT PERSON for communication from the family. You might set up and maintain a website where you can keep concerned friends and other family members apprised. Drs. Cynthia Moore and Paula Rauch (2010), in *Psycho-Oncology*, suggest that families with children designate a "Minister of Information" who will keep family and friends up-to-date. They write, "Frequent visitors, telephone calls, or reported inquiries from well-wishers about the parent's health while the child and parent are together can lead children to feel that their whole world is about cancer" (p. 529). They also suggest that families designate a "Captain of Kindness" to orchestrate help from others.

SUPPORT THE CAREGIVER. Remember that he will struggle, as well. He will have tremendous needs, both practical and emotional. Listen, empathize, provide feedback, offer to help, encourage—offer to help in the same ways you would for your friend. If he'd like, help him find a support group and offer to stay with your friend or the children (if applicable) while he attends the group sessions.

EMPHASIZE TO THE CAREGIVER the importance of taking breaks, and offer to stay with your friend so he can have some time for himself. Respite can be one of the most important gifts you can give the caregiver. Oftentimes, he will feel socially isolated and may suffer high levels of anxiety and depression. Cancer care professionals strongly urge caregivers to find ways to make time for themselves and, especially, to attend to their own physical needs—exercise, periods of relaxation, and so forth. Time away is not a luxury—it is a necessity. Many people with cancer point out that they, too, need time away from their caregivers!

TAKE SOME OF THE BURDEN off the caregiver.
Caregivers, especially spouses, will often try to handle everything themselves—around-the-clock care for the person with cancer, transportation to and from treatment, housework, insurance claims, cooking, laundry. It can't be done. There is always too much for one person to do. Offer to help by cooking, doing laundry, running errands, grocery shopping—whatever will be most helpful. If the caregiver has become totally overloaded, assist him in finding help. This could be assistance with practical matters: housecleaning, help with transportation, or caring for children. If you are good friends with the family and you feel comfortable doing so, you might ask him about counseling, if it seems that he is struggling. On the American Cancer Society's website (cancer. org), you can find a "Distress Checklist for Caregivers," which is designed to help caregivers gauge their own well-being. Many cancer clinics have a social worker who can find help for the caregiver if it's needed.

REMEMBER TO RECOGNIZE the caregiver's efforts. He needs to hear praise for what he does and acknowledgment from others that he, too, is suffering (Gilbar & Ben-Zur, 2002). Tell him that his efforts are seen and appreciated. Give him a card or gift. One woman was given a cappuccino maker as a gift by friends in recognition of all she had done. They realized how much she had sacrificed, too.

49

LET FAMILY MEMBERS KNOW that you are available to listen without judgment. Reassure them that you will keep your conversations confidential, and follow through on your word. They need release and validation of their feelings just as much as the person with cancer.

ASK HOW BEST TO HELP with childcare. Your friend's children and their welfare will be everything to her. Their needs will depend, of course, upon their ages and the family's particular circumstances. You might provide reliable transportation to and from school or afterschool activities, sporting events, or music lessons. If you're able, you could offer to watch her children during school breaks or summer vacation. Perhaps full-time childcare is not needed, but your friend could use some occasional down time. You might offer to take her children to the park every Saturday morning so she can rest. Depending on their ages, caring for the children might be most appropriate for those who have already established a familiar and long-term relationship with them. The children may have preferences, so do not be offended if they are more comfortable with other friends.

HELP SUPPORT THE CHILDREN as much as possible. The children may feel left out but have trouble expressing it directly. If you are close to the family, don't be afraid to step in and help support the children. Offer to drive them to their regular activities or lessons, if you are able to commit to a regular schedule. Help them with their homework. Assist with birthdays and holiday activities, or take them on outings. Keeping some sense of normalcy and routine is very important for children at all ages. Routine is important in giving them security.

LISTEN IF THE KIDS WANT TO TALK about their parent's illness, but don't push them to open up. You might offer to help find a professional or facilitated support group of other kids going through similar experiences. Many communities have support groups for children whose parents have cancer. Your friend's oncology clinic may be able to help with references. See the resource guide starting on page 79 for information on support groups for children.

51

GIVE THE CHILDREN gifts. Age-related gifts that provide entertainment are nice. Any gift, really, that you'd give the children for a special occasion would be enjoyed. Food treats are almost always welcome.

HELP YOUR FRIEND keep in touch with her children if she is away from them (while hospitalized, for example). Sometimes the vital need for connection between parent and child gets lost in the shuffle. If you are helping to provide childcare while the parent is hospitalized, help to enable frequent contact through Skype, FaceTime, regular phone calls, or in-person visits. Video or photograph the children on outings and share these moments with your friend.

DON'T...

DON'T GIVE THE CHILD INFORMATION that could distress him or her further. Remember how sensitive a child could be to anything mentioned about the ill parent. You'll definitely want to talk with the child's parents about how they would like you to approach the subject with their child. You'll want to abide by their wishes.

DON'T ACT AS A COUNSELOR for your friend's child. You can give him or her heaps of affection, be a good listener, bring gifts and treats, help with whatever needs come up, but don't take on the role of counselor.

CHAPTER 4

AFTER
TREATMENT
ENDS

The final day of my radiation treatment was much
the same as all the other days had been. The folks
at the radiation clinic kindly gave me the customary
end-of-treatment cake and took a Polaroid of me,
bald and smiling. Then I went home.

I was so tired by that time that it took a long
while to recognize that active treatment was
indeed "over." Though a party would have been
appreciated, I found that celebrating a few weeks
later worked best for me. It was then that it had
finally sunk in—I'd made it through!

My life didn't exactly pick up where it had left off
before my cancer diagnosis. At that time, I'd just
begun classes at Colorado State University to

complete work for a degree. The diagnosis certainly derailed those plans, and I found it difficult to regain my footing when treatment was over. I was very, very tired—and extremely anxious. Sometimes I felt as if my well-being—my life, really—depended solely upon the outcomes from follow-up visits with my oncologist. I was fortunate, though, in that my home life had gone relatively smoothly throughout my treatment and afterward. My daughter was married, and my son away at college. My husband, Jim, had continued to work throughout my treatment.

Even still, something was different. I didn't feel quite "fixed" in the way you might if you'd broken your ankle and gotten the cast removed. Indeed, something had changed.

Many might feel that a celebration is fitting when treatment ends. Your friend has indeed reached a milestone, but you'll need to be aware of her cues or simply ask her directly how and when she'd like to mark the occasion.

In some cases, this will be your friend's most challenging time in dealing with cancer. Now is the time when the real grief process begins. She has just been through an emotionally and physically grueling experience, one which has no doubt affected every aspect of her life. Energy levels and physical stamina are likely at their lowest point. The fatigue that has probably been wearing on your friend over the course of her treatment does not simply disappear, but can linger for some time after treatment ends. In fact, fatigue is the most common complaint in the first year after treatment (Baker, Denniston, Smith, & West, 2005). Cancer researcher Dr. Lillian Nail (2004) describes the feeling as, "My get up and go got up and went." Cancer-related fatigue can be debilitating and continues for months or even years after treatment ends in approximately one-third of people with cancer (Hofman, Ryan, Figueroa-Moseley, Jean-Pierre, & Morrow, 2007).

55

In 2004, the Livestrong Foundation conducted a large-scale survey of people who had undergone cancer treatment (Rechis & Boerner, 2010). The majority of the respondents were more than two years out from their diagnosis, and almost half of those were more than five years out. Some of the results may help you know what your friend could be going through: 72 percent had suffered depression as a result of their cancer, and 40 percent said that their lives were still consumed by cancer and related issues. Ten percent said they still had daily conversations about their cancer, 14 percent weekly, and 32 percent a few times per month. Many survivors five years out encounter very few problems, aside from the typical concerns that anyone—not just someone who's had cancer—would have (Ganz et al., 2002). But it's helpful to understand that cancer is not necessarily over when treatment ends, and for many survivors, distress can persist for some time after treatment. As my friend Ann pointed out, "There are some things from which you don't really ever recover."

More than 14 million people who have had cancer are living in the United States today—many of whom are at least five years out from diagnosis (DeSantis et al., 2014). Thanks to advances in early detection and treatments for cancer, cancer survivors are now living longer. People who have undergone cancer treatment often experience physical, emotional, psychological, and financial hardships as a result of their experiences. Many encounter obstacles, including difficulties getting quality health care after treatment. Some survivors even fit the criteria for a diagnosis of post-traumatic stress disorder.

As the population of cancer survivors and the meaning of survivorship have changed, the long-term effects of cancer and its treatment are being studied and considered more carefully by the medical establishment. There is still need for improvement, however, in how survivors are cared for in the long term.

Many people will expect your friend to be back to normal, to resume her "pre-cancer" family roles, and perhaps return to work after a long absence.

Your friend may feel hurried by circumstances (or by her own desire to get back to her pre-cancer life), but she will still need lots of time to adjust. It can take years for her to feel "normal" again, and many families (and patients) are unprepared for a long transition (National Cancer Institute, 2014). The idea of cancer survivors simply picking up where they left off does not match up to people's actual experiences. For most survivors, the experience of having cancer has changed their lives, and them, in lasting ways. In addition, the emotional recovery from a cancer crisis takes longer than the physical recovery—a fact that family and friends and even health care providers often fail to remember (Murphy, Morris, & Lange, 1997).

Jana Bolduan Lomax (personal communication, March 13, 2014), a clinical health psychologist, says, "After treatment ends, family and friends might think, 'It's over.' And they *want* it to be over. Yet, for their loved one with cancer, it's not. She may not want to bring up that she's still fatigued, that cancer is still of a part of her life every day— and always will be—that she is forever different in some way because of facing and surviving cancer."

57

The transition from patient to "healthy person" brings about an additional sense of insecurity and vulnerability. People who've had cancer report mixed feelings about the end of treatment, and for many it is a source of anxiety and worry. It is crucial for friends and family to try to understand this conflict.

For months, the person has been undergoing treatment for the cancer, an experience that, while arduous, is also reassuring. Something is being "done" to wipe out the cancer. There are regular check-ups with medical professionals and regular scans and blood tests to check the treatment's progress. The end of treatment can leave one feeling as if she has been abandoned by the doctors and nurses who have played such a large role in her life. One of my friends noted that she felt "tossed outside of the 'cancer culture'" that she had inhabited for so long and found it difficult to focus her life on something other than disease. "I had to learn that the world was bigger than 'Doctors' Lane,'" she said.

Often, people who finish treatment, having learned cancer's "lessons," are disillusioned when they re-enter their pre-cancer lives. Arlene Houldin (2000), in her book *Patients with Cancer*, cites a common experience of those who are newly out of treatment:

> *I expected all my family problems to vanish when treatment was over. I hoped the family learned, as I have come to learn, the preciousness of life and the stupidity of wasting energy bickering about trivial, inconsequential matters. But I was wrong and I am so disappointed. Not only are all the problems back, but I also feel completely alone now, because I no longer see these things as important and they do* (p. 36).

Fear that the cancer will return hits full force at the end of treatment. At this point, in fact, fears of recurrence are often at their highest. Of all the fears a person who has finished cancer treatment will face, more than anything, it's fear of recurrence. This never totally disappears. Fear of recurrence may last more than five years beyond the date of diagnosis and may be felt at nearly the same level of intensity as it was in the first five years (Koch, Jansen, Brenner, & Arndt, 2013).

The literature provides compelling evidence. In the Livestrong Foundation study cited earlier (Rechis & Boerner, 2010), fear of recurrence from cancer remained active in 66 percent of respondents. "How am I supposed to know if I have it again the second time around?" a friend once asked me. "I certainly had no clue the first time." This nagging anxiety can feel like constantly waiting for the other shoe to drop. Any time your friend has an unusual ache, an abnormal sensation, or a routine follow-up examination, she will be on edge—aware of what "could" happen.

My friend John's story is characteristic: About two years after he had a dime-sized melanoma surgically removed from his back, he found himself worrying about a new black spot he discovered under one of his fingernails. It was a Saturday, so he didn't think he could get an appointment with his dermatologist. That afternoon, he went to the grocery story and miraculously saw his doctor

59

poking around in the vegetable department. He rushed over, offered a hurried apology, and asked whether the dermatologist could take a quick look. The doctor sighed as though he'd seen this sort of behavior before, glanced at the finger, and asked whether John had banged his finger recently. He had. That was more than twenty years ago, and John laughs about it all the time now. But he didn't laugh then.

Even though researchers have found many signs of distress in those who are living with cancer, they also point out that some people ultimately find benefit in this experience. S. Leigh (1992) points out that along with the difficulties of survivorship, some do find a silver lining—termed "benefit-finding" in the scientific literature. A cancer diagnosis can cause a person to re-examine her priorities, pay more attention to personal relationships, become more empathetic toward others, and take better care of herself.

DO...

WHEN APPROPRIATE, CELEBRATE her completion of treatment in a way that is fitting, whether it be a small gathering, lunch out, or a big get-together. Now might be the time to send flowers or a houseplant for her living room or patio.

TAKE HER for an outdoor getaway. Time outdoors is a great way to acknowledge and celebrate this milestone in her cancer experience. It doesn't have to be elaborate. If she is just beginning to get some energy back, a short outing might be best. You might take a stroll around a lake, through a park, or in the foothills.

CONTINUE TO OFFER practical help and support in the ways you did during her treatment. Her energy levels will not be where they were before treatment. Her life will not be where it was before treatment. She will still appreciate help with housework and meals and other practical tasks. And she most certainly needs all the continued intricacies of friendship. Research has found that frequent visits with friends and family foster positive feelings and can form a fabric in which the person can thrive and feel a sense of belonging after treatment (Sapp et al., 2003).

SURPRISES OR GIFTS would still be welcome. It will take some time for her to get her footing. Little gifts or surprises will brighten her days.

JOIN HER IN ACTIVITIES she enjoyed before her diagnosis. Dr. Robert W. Lent (2007), a professor of counseling psychology at the University of Maryland, emphasizes that those who are adjusting to life after treatment should focus on enjoyable activities that may have been

61

difficult or impossible during treatment. Activities that include a social component and have an "outward focus" are especially good. "The importance of reentry, or increasing involvement, in valued life activities can probably not be overemphasized" (p. 242), Lent stresses.

HELP HER FIND TIMES to rest. If she has young children, offer to take them out while she takes a nap. Remind her teenager to turn down the loud music. If you can run an errand for her, shop for groceries, or pay bills, offer your help so she can take time for herself.

BE PATIENT WITH HER during anxious times. A level of uncertainty and fear will always be with her; try to be understanding of the complicated emotions of life after cancer. Routine follow-up appointments and tests are particularly anxiety provoking. Offer to accompany her to these appointments. Other triggers include anniversary dates or news about someone who has died of cancer. Let her know that you are always open to talk at these times.

BE PATIENT if your friend has trouble recalling things she would have at one time easily remembered. Chemotherapy can impair memory, attention, concentration, and mental processing speed, resulting in a real and diagnosable condition called "chemo brain."

One in four people with cancer has reported memory and attention problems following chemotherapy—sometimes lasting a short while, sometimes years (National Cancer Institute, 2014). In one study, breast cancer survivors exhibited cognitive deficits more than twenty years after chemotherapy (Koppelmans et al., 2012). Unfortunately, some may never regain full cognitive function (University of Texas MD Anderson Cancer Center, 2014). Someone I know well has chemo brain and says that it not only affects her intellectual life, but her social life as well. "I have to write down everything or it's gone from my mind. And what bothers me most is that I tend to repeat things over and over to my friends, with no awareness that I'm doing it. And things that my friends have told me—things that before cancer I would have remembered forever—are forgotten. It's really detrimental to friendships."

REMEMBER THAT SHE HAS UNDERGONE a life-changing event, which may have had short- or long-term side effects. Besides the possibility of chemo brain, these side effects can include fatigue, changed body image, low libido, wavering emotions, sleep issues, and pain. Some of these can be lessened or treated with medication or therapy, or will take time to fade away on their own. Many people who've had cancer continue speaking with members of a support group and are able to find the help and encouragement they need in that setting. Your friend may be so grateful to have gotten through treatment that she will consider these side effects minor inconveniences, but that may depend on the severity and nature of the changes.

OFFER TO BE her exercise buddy. Go walking with her, or bicycling, or on a short hike. Or join a fitness class with her, something you would both enjoy. Exercise has so many benefits for people who have completed cancer treatment. Most often, it's easier and more enjoyable to exercise with a friend. She will likely need to check with her doctor as to the right level of exercise for her. She may need to start out slowly and make some modifications. But the evidence linking physical activity with improved quality of life in those in treatment and after treatment "is incredibly strong," according to Dr. Rachel Ballard-Barbash from the National Cancer Institute (Phillips, 2010).

Along with all of the physical benefits, studies have shown that exercise can reduce cancer-related fatigue, decrease anxiety and depression, and improve self-esteem and mood in cancer survivors (Courneya et al., 2003; Schmitz et al., 2010). Other studies have shown that exercise after treatment can improve one's body image and reduce treatment-related pain (Irwin et al., 2013; Szabo, 2013).

DON'T...

DON'T PRETEND the cancer never occurred.
Some fear that mentioning their friend's cancer
will disrupt the healing process. However, she
needs acknowledgement of what she has been
through. On the other hand, she may be eager
to resume a more normal life as time passes
and she moves on from cancer treatment. Your
interactions might require some fine tuning during
her adjustment to life after active treatment.

**DON'T TRY TO RUSH YOUR FRIEND through
the recovery process.** Healing will take time.
People may want your friend to be okay, to be
"better," but it is important that she be given
the space and time she needs to recover. In the
book *What Helped Get Me Through*, Dr. Julie
Silver (2009), a Harvard-based physiatrist and
breast cancer survivor writes, "[H]ealing can take
months or years—even in someone who is very
dedicated to recovering as well as possible. This
is frustrating for many cancer survivors who want
to heal quickly and well. Healing is a process that
can be *facilitated* but not *rushed*. I think of this as
tempo gusto, a musical term that means 'at the
right speed'" (p. 271).

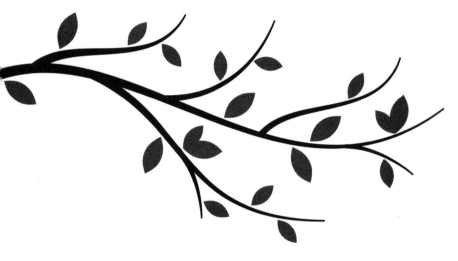

CHAPTER 5

IF A CURE IS NO LONGER POSSIBLE

In the many years since my treatment for cancer, I have shown "no evidence of disease." I'm extremely grateful. In these same years, however, I've occasionally learned that someone I knew from my support group, or perhaps met in the chemo room or the oncologist's waiting room, has succumbed to cancer.

It's always sobering to realize that not everyone survives a cancer diagnosis. In spite of the mighty will to live, a strong devotion to faith, careful adherence to a medical plan—in spite of everything.

My very personal experience was my mother's death from recurrent breast cancer in 2009. She was seventy-nine years old. Her first bout of breast cancer had occurred before she was forty, so her diagnosis, decades later, came as a shock, just as it does for most everyone diagnosed with cancer.

I saw the wide range of reactions to her advanced illness that I'd learned to expect—even the fear and avoidance. But my mother was much loved by her neighbors, former coworkers, and members of her church, and she had lots of close friends who supported her and gave her comfort. I saw once again how much difference the generosity and compassion of friends can make for someone with cancer. Kindness does indeed work wonders.

When treatment ends, sometimes the cancer will continue to grow. Your friend may try additional treatments, consult with other specialists, or—with great hope—participate in a clinical trial. Yet the cancer just keeps growing. When everything has been tried and there are no treatment options left, her doctor must deliver the news: There is nothing left to do. There is no cure.

These are probably the most difficult words ever to take in.

At this time, her journey takes her to a different road, one with lots of uncertainties and few signposts. Your friend will encounter peaks and valleys as she tries to navigate this road, but you can accompany her along the way.

There can be many phases in this stage. Some people are able to live for some time knowing that there will not be a cure for them. For others, the journey may be shorter. Your friend might be very active and functional when she receives the news. She may be weak and unable to get around at this point, or she may be somewhere between these phases.

Regardless of your friend's physical state, there are many things you still can do to help her and her family.

DO...

CONTINUE TO GIVE YOUR FRIEND the gift of your presence. Unfortunately, it is not uncommon for people to withdraw from someone they care about who is dying. Being with your friend will likely be difficult. It's scary. It's emotionally painful. It's heartbreaking. You'll need to draw on all of your inner strength to serve as a source of strength for her. Just don't abandon her.

Remember that your friend also may be feeling a sense of loss as she transitions from active treatment and no longer feels the support or presence of her medical team. Vanessa Wolfe (personal communication, April 5, 2014), a hospice nurse in northern Colorado, notes that people with cancer can often feel a great loss when they are no longer connected to this vital support system. "For a long while, they've been cared for by doctors, nurses, social workers, and others who have focused on their treatment. Chances are that they've formed a bond with many of them. Now, that entire system may be gone. It can be a huge adjustment."

REALIZE THAT TALKING about this time in your friend's life is healthy. You'll need to follow her lead and that of her family, of course. Talking about dying is difficult. But it is vital for family members and loved ones to be open and honest about what's happening. We may believe we're protecting our loved one who's ill by avoiding discussion of anything upsetting, but this leads to isolation for the person with cancer and her surrounding loved ones. Maggie Callanan (2008), a long-time hospice nurse and author, calls this "the 'Pink-hippopotamus-in-the-tutu syndrome…' The pink hippo—the reality of dying—sits right in the middle of the room. Everyone sees it and walks around it, but no one mentions it, pretending it's not there. The atmosphere around the dying person becomes artificial…" (p. 18).

SUPPORT HER in her wishes. These could be anything. If she's able, she may decide to take that trip to Alaska she always talked about. She may want to track down a relative with whom she's been out of touch. It could be as simple as wanting to go out to eat more often. The possibilities, and the fulfillment of her wishes, will naturally depend upon her health. But help her in whatever way you can.

SUPPORT HER DECISIONS, as well. These decisions might involve day-to-day matters or something much more significant. She and her family will have many decisions to make, both large and small. Don't question her choices.

One choice your friend will likely be given by her doctor, when there is no longer hope for a cure, is whether or when to enter hospice care. Although each hospice care organization in the United States might operate a little bit differently, they all focus on quality of life rather than length of life. And they do so in a holistic manner, meaning they care for the whole person, providing medical services as they also attend to the person's emotional, social, and spiritual well-being. In addition, they provide a great deal of support for the family.

Those who are unfamiliar with the goals of hospice care might perceive that the person has "given up" by entering hospice. Vanessa Wolfe says she frequently hears this misconception. But people who enter hospice care have not given up, they have only changed their focus: to being cared for rather than being cured. Even with their prognoses, she says, they're still living their lives, as comfortably as possible.

RECOGNIZE THAT COPING STYLES often remain consistent throughout one's life. Her method of dealing with stress or difficulties will not suddenly change because she's been told she is dying. Callanan describes a pattern of behavior well known

71

to those who work with the dying and their families: "People die as they live—intensified" (p. 135). Quiet people become quieter; busy people get busier. Callanan recommends that you think about how the person has typically reacted to stress in her life. By anticipating what is to come, it may be easier to understand her reactions and behavior.

LISTENING IS MORE IMPORTANT now than ever. It is not just listening that is important, but the way in which you listen. Dr. Robert Buckman and coauthors (1992), in *I Don't Know What to Say: How to Help and Support Someone Who Is Dying*, devote an entire chapter to "sensitive listening." Among their suggestions: Keep your eyes on the same level as hers, within a comfortable distance, and maintain a calm, unrushed demeanor. Good listening is more than just sitting there like a running tape recorder. Demonstrate that you are hearing and listening, with an affirming nod of the head or a gentle smile. Nonverbal communication often says as much or more as verbal communication.

TELL HER THE WAYS that she has graced your life. Reminisce about things you've done together. Do this often. You might consider writing her a letter expressing your gratitude. Many people don't realize how meaningful a heartfelt letter can be— even more so than engaging with a friend, which may require more energy than she has to spare.

APPRECIATE THE IMPORTANCE spirituality may play at this stage. Spirituality often intensifies in this stage of life, particularly if it was already an important part of her life. Callanan writes, "Spirituality infuses every aspect of our lives but [can] intensif[y] greatly as death approaches, even for those who have strayed from their original faith. It is most often our spiritual beliefs that give strength, meaning, and direction during these ultimately challenging life events" (p. 176). Most spiritual belief systems have writings on death and dying that can be very helpful. Ask your friend whether she would like books or CDs regarding death and dying. However, be sensitive if spirituality has not been part of your friendship; especially in this stage of life, the personal nature of spirituality makes it a subject you should approach with care.

73

HELP HER FINISH THINGS she doesn't want to leave undone. Perhaps you can help her finish a family photo album, buy Christmas or birthday presents, compose letters to children or other family members, or help write her life story. Help her prioritize what's most important to do and what doesn't really need to be done—such as cleaning out a closet, unless that's really important to her. Don't try to tell her what she needs or wants.

TAPE THE CARDS AND NOTES she has received to the ceiling over her bed so she can see them while she's lying down.

HELP HER GET COMFORTABLE. Fluff her pillows, make sure her water glass is easy to reach, and ensure that she has food she likes and can eat. Try not to make her ask for everything she needs. Try to anticipate her needs without making her crazy.

READ TO HER; play soft music. Or sit with her even if she dozes. Just having someone there can be very comforting.

BE AWARE OF HER FAMILY'S NEEDS, especially as these needs relate to time with their loved one. As the cancer continues to advance and patients become weaker, they will be less engaged in the environment around them. They begin to pull away or withdraw, and quality time with the family will become more limited. Some families will want to spend this time alone with their loved one without friends around. Some even post Do Not Disturb signs. Respect their wishes, and do not visit unannounced. Remember that there are other ways to show your love and support without being physically present. You might leave a gift card at the door or write a kind note to your friend that the family can read to her.

CELEBRATE HER LIFE. Be grateful for your friendship. Keep her loved ones in your thoughts. Continue, always, to be kind. In the end, it is kindness that gets us through.

AMERICAN CANCER SOCIETY

CANCER IS
SO LIMITED

They've sentenced you with invisible cells that
secret themselves deep in body recesses and multiply:
lymphatic assault on vital functions.

Can cancer conquer you?
I doubt it, for the strengths I see in you have
nothing to do with cells and blood and muscle.

For cancer is so limited—
It cannot cripple love.
It cannot shatter hope.
It cannot corrode faith.
It cannot eat away peace.
It cannot destroy confidence.
It cannot kill friendship.
It cannot shut out memories.
It cannot silence courage.
It cannot invade the soul.
It cannot reduce eternal life.
It cannot quench the spirit.
It cannot cancel Resurrection.

Can cancer conquer you?
I doubt it, for the strengths I see in you have
nothing to do with cells and blood and muscle.

RESOURCE GUIDE

AMERICAN CANCER SOCIETY SUPPORT PROGRAMS AND SERVICES

American Cancer Society
Toll-free Line: 800-227-2345
Website: www.cancer.org

The American Cancer Society provides educational materials, information, and patient services to help people with cancer and their loved ones understand cancer, manage their lives through treatment and recovery, and find the emotional support they need. A comprehensive resource for all your cancer-related questions, the Society can also put you in touch with community resources in your area.

American Cancer Society Cancer Survivors Network® is an online community of cancer survivors, families, and friends who have been touched by cancer and want to share their experiences, strength, and hope. Visit www. acscsn.org to learn more.

American Cancer Society Clinical Trials Matching Service is a free, confidential program that helps patients, their families, and health care workers find cancer clinical trials most appropriate to a patient's medical and personal situation. For information, go to cancer.org and click on "Treatment Tools" or call a clinical trial specialist at 800-303-5691.

American Cancer Society Patient Navigator Program helps patients, families, and caregivers navigate the many systems needed during the cancer journey. Trained patient navigators at cancer treatment centers link those dealing with cancer to needed programs and resources.

Hope Lodge® communities offer cancer patients and their families a free, temporary place to stay when their best hope for effective treatment may be in another city. Accommodations and eligibility requirements may vary by location, and room availability is first come, first served.

Look Good Feel Better® is a free, community-based program that teaches beauty techniques to female cancer patients to help them manage the appearance-related side effects of cancer treatment. For more information, visit www.lookgoodfeelbetter.org.

Reach To Recovery® helps people (female and male) cope with their breast cancer experience. Reach To Recovery volunteers, themselves breast cancer survivors, offer understanding, support, and hope.

Road To Recovery® provides transportation to and from treatment for people who have cancer who do not have a ride or are unable to drive themselves. Volunteer drivers donate their time and the use of their cars.

"tlc" Tender Loving Care is the American Cancer Society's catalog and magazine for women with cancer. It offers helpful articles and a line of products such as wigs, hairpieces, hats, turbans, breast forms, mastectomy bras, and swimwear. To order products or catalogs, call 800-850-9445, or visit *tlc* online at www.tlcdirect.org.

GENERAL CANCER INFORMATION AND SUPPORT

CancerCare, Inc.
Toll-free Line: 800-813-HOPE (800-813-4673)
Website: www.cancercare.org

CancerCare is a nonprofit social service agency that provides counseling and guidance to help cancer patients and their families and friends cope with the impact of cancer. CancerCare offers support groups; teleconferences for patients, friends, and family members; workshops, seminars, and clinics; information on cancer, treatment, and clinical trials; and publications. CancerCare also provides a financial assistance program in New Jersey, New York, and Connecticut.

Cancer Connection
Telephone: 413-586-1642
Website: www.cancer-connection.org

Cancer Connection is a community-based nonprofit organization. It offers a haven where people living with cancer, their families, and their caregivers can learn to cope with their changed lives and bodies and their emotional challenges.

Cancer Hope Network
Toll-free Line: 800-552-4366
Website: www.cancerhopenetwork.org

Cancer Hope Network is a nonprofit organization that provides free and confidential one-on-one support to cancer patients and their families. Their core offering is to match cancer patients or family members with trained volunteers who have undergone and recovered from a similar cancer experience.

Cancer Support Community
Toll-free Line: 888-793-9355
Website: www.cancersupportcommunity.org

The Cancer Support Community provides emotional and social support through a network of local affiliates and satellite locations. It also offers a "Create Your Own Webpage" feature to allow users to post updates, create a helping calendar, and post financial needs.

4th Angel Patient and Mentoring Program
Toll-free Line: 866-520-3197
Website: www.4thangel.org

The 4th Angel Mentoring Program provides free and confidential telephone or e-mail support to cancer patients and their caregivers. Trained mentors, who are cancer survivors themselves or have been a caregiver to a cancer patient, offer guidance and support.

Friend for Life Cancer Support Network

Toll-free Line: 866-374-3634
Website: www.friend4life.org

Friend for Life Cancer Support Network is a network of cancer survivors who provide free one-on-one support to cancer patients and their loved ones.

Imerman Angels
Toll-free Line: 877-274-5529
Website: www.imermanangels.org

Imerman Angels is an organization that enables one-on-one support among cancer patients, survivors, and caregivers. This matching service is free and can help anyone touched by a cancer experience.

LIVESTRONG Survivor Care Program
Toll-free Line: 855-220-7777
Website: www.livestrong.org

The LIVESTRONG Survivor Care Program helps anyone affected by cancer. It helps people understand their options and what to expect. One-on-one support is provided along the way.

National Cancer Institute
Toll-free Line: 800-4-CANCER (800-422-6237)
TTY: 800-332-8615
Website: www.cancer.gov

The National Cancer Institute (NCI) provides information on cancer research, diagnosis, and treatment to patients and health care providers. Callers are automatically connected to the office serving their region. The service offers free publications and the opportunity to speak directly with a cancer specialist who can provide information on treatment and make appropriate referrals. NCI also offers a comprehensive database, "National Organizations That Offer Cancer-Related Support Services."

PRACTICAL, HOUSEHOLD, AND FINANCIAL ASSISTANCE*

The Assistance Fund
Toll-free Line: 855-845-3663
Website: www.assistfund.org

The Assistance Fund offers financial support to chronically ill individuals to help pay for prescription medications or monthly health insurance premiums.

Cancer Financial Assistance Coalition (CFAC)
Website: www.cancerfac.org

CFAC is a coalition of financial assistance organizations joining forces to help limit financial challenges for cancer patients. Its website includes a database of organizations that provide financial assistance.

*Patients may be required to satisfy certain criteria to be eligible for assistance.

CaringBridge.org
Telephone: 651-789-2300
Website: www.caringbridge.org

CaringBridge provides free websites to connect people experiencing significant health challenges with their family and friends. Websites offer a personal and private space to communicate and show support.

Cleaning for a Reason
Toll-free Line: 877-337-3348
Website: www.cleaningforareason.org

Cleaning for a Reason is a nonprofit organization that offers professional housecleaning services to help women undergoing treatment for any type of cancer.

Corporate Angel Network
Toll-free Line: 914-328-1313
Website: www.corpangelnetwork.org

The Corporate Angel Network arranges over 2,500 free flights per year on corporate jets for cancer patients, bone marrow donors, and bone marrow recipients who are able to walk up and down the steps to a private plane without assistance and do not require oxygen, IV, or any other form of life support during the flight.

Healthcare Hospitality Network
Toll-free Line: 800-542-9730
Website: www.hhnetwork.org

The Healthcare Hospitality Network is an association of nonprofit organizations that provide lodging and support services to patients, families, and their loved ones who are receiving medical treatment far from home.

Meal Train
Website: www.mealtrain.com

Meal Train is a free website that simplifies the organization of giving and receiving meals. The site allows recipients to share food preferences, preferred meal times, and available days.

MedGift

Website: www.medgift.com

MedGift offers free, private websites for people dealing with difficult medical situations. Sites include calendar and fundraising components, in addition to a place for status updates.

My Lifeline

Website: www.mylifeline.org

Mylifeline.org offers free, private patient websites for people affected by cancer. Sites include calendar and fundraising components, as well as journal features that allow friends and family to follow the patient's journey.

National Patient Travel Center

Toll-free Line: 800-296-1217
Website: www.patienttravel.org

The National Patient Travel Center provides information about all forms of charitable, long-distance medical transportation and provides referrals to other sources that can help.

NeedyMeds

Toll-free Line: 800-503-6897
Website: www.needymeds.org

NeedyMeds is an online resource of programs that provide assistance to people who are unable to afford their medications and health care costs. These programs make drugs available for free or at low cost to patients who are uninsured or underinsured.

Partnership for Prescription Assistance

Website: www.pparx.org

The Partnership for Prescription Assistance helps qualifying patients without prescription drug coverage get needed medicines. The organization provides a Directory of Prescription Drug Patient Assistance Programs that contains information about how to make a request for assistance, what prescription medicines are covered, and basic eligibility criteria.

Patient Advocate Foundation Co-Pay Relief Program
Toll-free Line: 866-512-3861
Website: www.copays.org

The Patient Advocate Foundation's Co-Pay Relief Program provides co-payment assistance to insured Americans who financially and medically qualify.

Patient Resource LLC
Toll-free Line: 800-497-7530
Website: www.patientresource.com

Patient Resource LLC provides comprehensive, easy-to-understand, up-to-date guides to treatment and facilities for people struggling with life-altering diseases. Information is free and offered online and in printed publications. They have an extensive list of organizations that offer financial assistance for cancer-related expenses, including childcare, equipment and supplies, home health care, housing during treatment, prescriptions, and transportation.

CAREGIVERS RESOURCES

Caregiving.com
Website: www.caregiving.com

Caregiving.com provides practical information on being a caregiver, managing the stress of caregiving, and solutions for caregiving situations. The website features the blogs of family caregivers, weekly words of comfort, weekly self-care plans, weekly chats, a Community Caregiving Journal, free webinars, and online support groups.

Family Caregiver Alliance
Toll-free Line: 800-445-8106
Website: www.caregiver.org

The Family Caregiver Alliance offers programs at the national, state, and local level to support and sustain caregivers. The website contains fact sheets, online support groups, newsletters, and links to other resources.

RESOURCES FOR CHILDREN, ADOLESCENTS, AND YOUNG ADULTS

Camp Kesem
Telephone: 260-225-3736
Website: www.campkesem.org

Camp Kesem is a week-long summer camp for kids with a parent who has (or had) cancer. The camps are free and provide the campers with extra attention and support through camp activities like sports, arts and crafts, and drama, as well as "Cabin Chats" with fellow campers and counselors.

Cancercare for Kids
Toll-free Line: 800-813-HOPE (800-813-4673)
Website: www.cancercareforkids.org/tagged/children

Cancercare for Kids is an online support program for teens with a parent, sibling, or other family member who has cancer. The toll-free line is also for anyone who has cancer or has a loved one with cancer.

Cancer in the Family Relief Fund
Telephone: 415-887-8932
Website: www.cancerfamilyrelieffund.org

Cancer in the Family Relief Fund facilitates grants to children whose parent or guardian is struggling with a diagnosis of cancer. These grants support children's extracurricular activities so that they may feel some sense of normalcy as their parent focuses on treatment and recovery.

Cancer Really Sucks
Website: www.cancerreallysucks.org

Cancer Really Sucks is an Internet-only resource designed for teens by teens who have loved ones facing cancer.

CLIMB®
Telephone: 303-322-1202
Website: www.childrenstreehousefdn.org

CLIMB® (Children's Lives Include Moments of Bravery) is a support group program for children of adult cancer patients. CLIMB helps normalize feelings of sadness, anxiety, fear, and anger, while helping improve communication between children and their parents.

KidsCope
Website: www.kidscope.org

KidsCope is an Internet-only resource for children and families. Its mission is to help children and families understand the effects of cancer or chemotherapy on a loved one, provide suggestions for coping, and develop innovative programs and materials that communicate a message of hope.

Kids Konnected
Toll-free Line: 800-899-2866
Website: www.kidskonnected.org

Kids Konnected offers groups and programs for children who have a parent with cancer. It provides information, referrals to local services, a newsletter, and grief workshops.

Planet Cancer
Telephone: 512-452-9010
Website: myplanet.planetcancer.org

Planet Cancer is an international community of support and advocacy for young adults with cancer in their twenties and thirties.

REFERENCE LIST

INTRODUCTION

Williams, T. T. (1991). *Refuge: An unnatural history of family and place*. New York, NY: Vintage Books.

CHAPTER 1

American Cancer Society. (2014). *Cancer information on the Internet*. Retrieved July 2, 2014, from http://www.cancer.org/cancer/cancerbasics/cancer-information-on-the-internet.

Frank, A. W. (2002). *At the will of the body: Reflections on illness*. New York, NY: Houghton Mifflin.

Gilbar, O., & Ben-Zur, H. (2002). *Cancer and the family caregiver: Distress and coping*. Springfield, IL: Charles C Thomas.

Granet, R. (2001). *Surviving cancer emotionally: Learning how to heal*. New York, NY: John Wiley & Sons.

Grange, C. M., Matsuyama, R. K., Ingram, K. M., Lyckholm, L. J., & Smith, T. J. (2008). Identifying supportive and unsupportive responses of others: Perspectives of African American and Caucasian cancer patients. *Journal of Psychosocial Oncology*, 26(1), 81–99.

Helgeson, V. S., & Cohen, S. (1996). Social support and adjustment to cancer: Reconciling descriptive, correlational, and intervention research. *Health Psychology*, 15(2), 135–148.

Houldin, A. D. (2000). *Patients with cancer: Understanding the psychological pain*. Philadelphia, PA: Lippincott Williams & Wilkins.

Keitel M. A., & Kopala, M. (2000). *Counseling women with breast cancer: A guide for professionals*. Thousand Oaks, CA: Sage Publications: 45.

Madsen, S. (2014, January 28). Arm's length: The distance between friendship and cancer. Article posted to http://www.huffingtonpost.com/stephaniemadsen/arms-length-the-distance-_b_4677828.html.

Mastrovito, R., Moynihan, R., & Parsonnet, L. (1989). Self-help and mutual support programs. In J. C. Holland & J. H. Rowland (Eds.), *Handbook of psychooncology:*

Psychological care of the patient with cancer (p. 504). New York, NY: Oxford University Press.

Matthews, B. A., Baker, F., & Spillers, R. L. (2004). Oncology professionals and patient requests for cancer support services. *Supportive Care in Cancer*, 12(10), 731–738.

Nouwen, H. J. M. (1974). *Out of solitude: Three meditations on the Christian life.* Notre Dame, IN: Ave Maria Press.

Peters-Golden, H. (1982). Breast cancer: Varied perceptions of social support in the illness experience. *Social Science & Medicine*,16(4), 483–491.

Puchalski, C. M. (2012). Spirituality in the cancer trajectory. *Annals of Oncology.* 23 Suppl 3, 49–55. doi: 10.1093/annonc/mds088.

Remen, R. N. (1997). *Kitchen table wisdom: Stories that heal.* New York, NY: Riverhead Books.

Sherman, D. (2014, January 22). Cancer wrecks your body, even some friendships. Message posted to http://blogs.reuters.com/cancer-in-context/2014/01/22/cancer-wrecks-your-body-even-some-friendships/.

Willis, J., & CancerCare, Inc. (2001). *The cancer patient's workbook: Everything you need to stay organized and informed.* New York: Dorling Kindersley Publishing.

CHAPTER 2

Cantor, R. C. (1978). *And a time to live: Toward emotional well-being during the crisis of cancer.* New York, NY: Harper & Row.

Cosmetic Executive Women Foundation. (2014). *How to be an effective "point person."* Retrieved July 1, 2014 from http://www.cancerandcareers.org/en/coworkers/How-to-be-an-Effective-Point-Person.

Grange, C. M., Matsuyama, R. K., Ingram, K. M., Lyckholm, L. J., & Smith, T. J. (2008). Identifying supportive and unsupportive responses of others: Perspectives of African American and Caucasian cancer patients. *Journal of Psychosocial Oncology*, 26(1), 81–99.

The Henry J. Kaiser Family Foundation, Harvard School of Public Health, *USA Today.* (2006, November). National survey of households affected by cancer. Menlo Park, CA; The Henry J. Kaiser Family Foundation.

Institute of Medicine Committee on Psychosocial Services to Cancer Patients / Families in a Community Setting. (2008). Adler NE, Page AEK, (Eds.). *Cancer care for the whole patient: Meeting psychosocial health needs.* Washington, DC: National Academies Press.

Longaker, C. (1997). *Facing death and finding hope: A guide to the emotional and spiritual care of the dying* (pp. 16–22). New York, NY: Doubleday.

Matthews, B. A., Baker, F., & Spillers, R. L. (2004). Oncology professionals and patient requests for cancer support services. *Supportive Care in Cancer*, 12(10), 731–738.

Peters-Golden, H. (1982). Breast cancer: Varied perceptions of social support in the illness experience. *Social Science & Medicine*,16(4), 483–491.

Roth, D. S. (2003). *An ovarian cancer companion*. Burnstown, Ontario: General Store Publishing House.

Rowland, J. H. (1989). Developmental stage and adaptation: Adult model. In J. C. Holland & J. H. Rowland (Eds.), *Handbook of psychooncology: Psychological care of the patient with cancer* (p. 36). New York, NY: Oxford University Press.

Silver, J. K. (Ed.). (2009). *What helped get me through: Cancer survivors share wisdom and hope*. Atlanta, GA: American Cancer Society.

Sprah, L., & Sostaric, M. (2004). Psychosocial coping strategies in cancer patients. *Radiology and Oncology*, 38(1), 35–42.

Thiboldeaux, K., Golant, M., & Cancer Support Community. (2012). *Reclaiming your life after diagnosis: The cancer support community handbook*. Dallas, TX: BenBella Books.

Weisman, A. D., & Worden, J. W. (1976-1977). The existential plight in cancer: Significance of the first 100 days. *The International Journal of Psychiatry in Medicine*, 7(1), 1–15.

Granet, R. (2001). *Surviving cancer emotionally: Learning how to heal.* New York, NY: John Wiley & Sons.

Montada, L., Filipp, S-H., & Lerner, M. J. (Eds.). (1992). *Life crises and experiences of loss in adulthood.* Abingdon, Oxon: Routledge.

Moore, C. W., & Rauch, P. K. (2010). Addressing the needs of children when a parent has cancer. In J. C. Holland, W. S. Breitbart, P. B. Jacobsen, M. S. Lederberg, M. J. Loscalzo, & R. McCorkle (Eds.), *Psycho-Oncology* (2nd ed.) (p. 529). New York, NY: Oxford University Press.

Northouse, L. L., Mood, D., Templin, T., Mellon, S., & George, T. (2000). Couples' patterns of adjustment to colon cancer. *Social Science & Medicine*, 50(2), 271–284.

Rait, D., & Lederberg, M. (1989). The family of the cancer patient. In J. C. Holland & J. H. Rowland. (Eds.). *Handbook of psychooncology: Psychological care of the patient with cancer* (p. 590). New York, NY: Oxford University Press.

Yabroff, K. R., & Kim, Y. (2009). Time costs associated with informal caregiving for cancer survivors. *Cancer*, 115(18), 4362–4373.

CHAPTER 4

Baker, F., Denniston, M., Smith, T., & West, M. M. (2005). Adult cancer survivors: How are they faring? *Cancer*, 104(11 Suppl), 2565–2576.

Courneya, K. S., Mackey, J. R., Bell, G. J., Jones, L. W., Field, C. J., & Fairey, A. S. (2003). Randomized controlled trial of exercise training in postmenopausal breast cancer survivors: Cardiopulmonary and quality of life outcomes. *Journal of Clinical Oncology*, 21(9), 1660–1668.

DeSantis, C. E., Lin, C. C., Mariotto, A. B., Siegel, R. L., Stein, K. D., Kramer, J. L., Alteri, R., Robbins, A. S., & Jemal, A. (2014). Cancer treatment and survivorship statistics, 2014. *CA: A Cancer Journal for Clinicians*, 64, 252–271. doi: 10.3322/caac.21235.

Ganz, P. A., Desmond, K. A., Leedham, B., Rowland, J. H., Meyerowitz, B. E., & Belin, T. R. (2002). Quality of life in long-term, disease-free survivors of breast cancer: A follow-up study. *Journal of the National Cancer Institute*, 94(1), 39–49.

Erratum in *Journal of the National Cancer Institute*, 94(6), 463.

Hofman, M., Ryan, J. L., Figueroa-Moseley, C. D., Jean-Pierre, P., & Morrow, G. R. (2007). Cancer-related fatigue: The scale of the problem. *The Oncologist*, 12(Suppl 1), 4–10.

Houldin, A. D. (2000). *Patients with cancer: Understanding the psychological pain.* Philadelphia, PA: Lippincott Williams & Wilkins.

Irwin, M., Cartmel, B., Gross, C., Ercolano, E., Fiellin, M., Capozza, S., Rothbard, M., Zhou, Y., Harrigan, M., Sanft, T., Schmitz, K., Neogi, T., Hershman, D., & Ligibel, J. Randomized trial of exercise vs. usual care on aromatase inhibitor-associated arthralgias in women with breast cancer. Paper presented at 36th Annual San Antonio Breast Cancer Symposium in December 2013, San Antonio, TX.

Koch, L., Jansen, L., Brenner, H., & Arndt, V. (2013). Fear of recurrence and disease progression in long-term (≥ 5 years) cancer survivors—a systematic review of quantitative studies. *Psychooncology*, 22(1), 1–11. doi: 10.1002/pon.3022.

Koppelmans, V., Breteler, M. M., Boogerd, W., Seynaeve, C., Gundy, C., & Schagen, S. B. (2012). Neuropsychological performance in survivors of breast cancer more than 20 years after adjuvant chemotherapy. *Journal of Clinical Oncology*, 30(10), 1080–1086. doi: 10.1200/JCO.2011.37.0189.

Leigh, S. (1992). Myths, monsters, and magic: Personal perspectives and professional challenges of survival. *Oncology Nursing Forum*, 19(10), 1475–1480.

Lent, R. W. (2007). Restoring emotional well-being: A model. In M. Feuerstein (Ed.), *Handbook of Cancer Survivorship* (p. 242). New York, NY: Springer.

Murphy, G., Morris, L. B., & Lange, D. (1997). *Informed decisions: The complete book of cancer diagnosis, treatment, and recovery.* Atlanta, GA: American Cancer Society.

Nail, L. M. (2004). My get up and go got up and went: Fatigue in people with cancer. *Journal of the National Cancer Institute Monographs*, (32), 72–75.

National Cancer Institute. (2014, May). *Facing forward: Life after cancer treatment.* Bethesda, MD: National Institutes of Health. NIH Publication No. 14-2424.

Phillips, C. (2010, June 29). Guidelines urge exercise for cancer patients, survivors. *NCI Cancer Bulletin.* Retrieved July 2, 2014 from http://www.cancer.gov/ncicancerbulletin/062910/page5.

Rechis, R., Boerner, L. (2010, June). How cancer has affected post-treatment survivors: A Livestrong report. Austin, TX; Livestrong Foundation.

Sapp, A. L., Trentham-Dietz, A., Newcomb, P. A., Hampton, J. M., Moinpour, C. M., & Remington, P. L. (2003). Social networks and quality of life among female long-term colorectal cancer survivors. *Cancer*, 98(8), 1749–1758.

Schmitz, K. H., Courneya, K. S., Matthews, C., Demark-Wahnefried, W., Galvão, D. A., Pinto, B. M., Irwin, M. L., Wolin, K. Y., Segal, R. J., Lucia, A., Schneider, C. M., von Gruenigen, V. E., Schwartz, A. L., & American College of Sports Medicine. (2010). American College of Sports Medicine roundtable on exercise guidelines for cancer survivors. *Medicine & Science in Sports & Exercise*, 42(7), 1409–1426. doi: 10.1249/MSS.0b013e3181e0c112.

Erratum in *Medicine & Science in Sports & Exercise*. 2011, 43(1), 195.

Silver, J. K. (Ed.). (2009). *What helped get me through: Cancer survivors share wisdom and hope*. Atlanta, GA: American Cancer Society.

Szabo, L. (2013, December 12). Exercise can ease pain from breast cancer drugs. *USA Today*. Retrieved from http://www.usatoday.com/story/news/nation/2013/12/12/exercise-can-ease-treatment-related-pain-in-breast-cancer/3983729/.

University of Texas MD Anderson Cancer Center. (2014). Chemobrain. Retrieved from http://www.mdanderson.org/patient-and-cancer-information/cancer-information/cancer-topics/dealing-with-cancer-treatment/chemobrain/index.html.

CHAPTER 5

Buckman, R., Gallop, R., & Martin, J. (1992). *I don't know what to say: How to help and support someone who is dying*. New York, NY: Vintage Books.

Callanan, M. (2008). *Final journeys: A practical guide to bringing care and comfort at the end of life*. New York, NY: Bantam.

INDEX

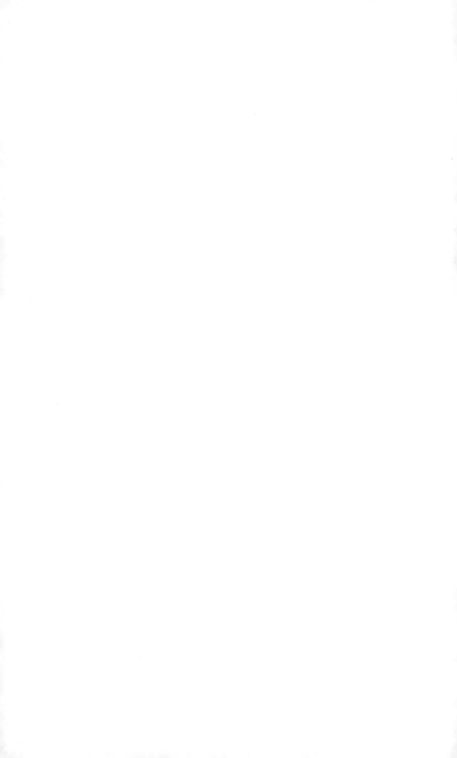

ABOUT THE
AUTHOR

Colleen Dolan Fullbright is a writer, journalist, educator, and breast cancer survivor. After her cancer diagnosis in 2000, she realized what a vital and uplifting part friends and family could play in one's cancer journey. A lifelong resident of Colorado, she lives in Fort Collins, with her husband, Jim. They have two children, six grandchildren, and one great-grandchild.

FOR CHILDREN

And Still They Bloom: A Family's Journey of Loss and Healing

Because… Someone I Love Has Cancer

Get Better! Communication Cards for Kids & Adults

Imagine What's Possible: Use the Power of Your Mind to Take Control of Your Life During Cancer

Let My Colors Out

The Long and the Short of It: A Tale About Hair

Mom and the Polka-Dot Boo-Boo

Nana, What's Cancer?

No Thanks, but I'd Love to Dance: Choosing to Live Smoke Free

Our Dad Is Getting Better

Our Mom Has Cancer

Our Mom Is Getting Better

What's Up with Bridget's Mom? Medikidz Explain Breast Cancer

What's Up with Tiffany's Dad? Medikidz Explain Melanoma

PREVENTION

The Great American Eat-Right Cookbook

Kicking Butts: Quit Smoking and Take Charge of Your Health, Second Edition

Maya's Secrets: Delightful Latin Dishes for a Healthier You

Visit **cancer.org/bookstore** for a full listing of books published by the American Cancer Society.